Joerg Traub

Intraoperative Imaging and Navigation

Joerg Traub

Intraoperative Imaging and Navigation

New Concepts for Design and Workflow Driven Evaluation of Computer Assisted Surgery Solutions

Südwestdeutscher Verlag für Hochschulschriften

Impressum/Imprint (nur für Deutschland/only for Germany)
Bibliografische Information der Deutschen Nationalbibliothek: Die Deutsche Nationalbibliothek verzeichnet diese Publikation in der Deutschen Nationalbibliografie; detaillierte bibliografische Daten sind im Internet über http://dnb.d-nb.de abrufbar.

Alle in diesem Buch genannten Marken und Produktnamen unterliegen warenzeichen-, marken- oder patentrechtlichem Schutz bzw. sind Warenzeichen oder eingetragene Warenzeichen der jeweiligen Inhaber. Die Wiedergabe von Marken, Produktnamen, Gebrauchsnamen, Handelsnamen, Warenbezeichnungen u.s.w. in diesem Werk berechtigt auch ohne besondere Kennzeichnung nicht zu der Annahme, dass solche Namen im Sinne der Warenzeichen- und Markenschutzgesetzgebung als frei zu betrachten wären und daher von jedermann benutzt werden dürften.

Verlag: Südwestdeutscher Verlag für Hochschulschriften GmbH & Co. KG
Dudweiler Landstr. 99, 66123 Saarbrücken, Deutschland
Telefon +49 681 37 20 271-1, Telefax +49 681 37 20 271-0
Email: info@svh-verlag.de

Approved by: München, TU, Diss, 2008

Herstellung in Deutschland:
Schaltungsdienst Lange o.H.G., Berlin
Books on Demand GmbH, Norderstedt
Reha GmbH, Saarbrücken
Amazon Distribution GmbH, Leipzig
ISBN: 978-3-8381-1203-9

Imprint (only for USA, GB)
Bibliographic information published by the Deutsche Nationalbibliothek: The Deutsche Nationalbibliothek lists this publication in the Deutsche Nationalbibliografie; detailed bibliographic data are available in the Internet at http://dnb.d-nb.de.

Any brand names and product names mentioned in this book are subject to trademark, brand or patent protection and are trademarks or registered trademarks of their respective holders. The use of brand names, product names, common names, trade names, product descriptions etc. even without a particular marking in this works is in no way to be construed to mean that such names may be regarded as unrestricted in respect of trademark and brand protection legislation and could thus be used by anyone.

Publisher: Südwestdeutscher Verlag für Hochschulschriften GmbH & Co. KG
Dudweiler Landstr. 99, 66123 Saarbrücken, Germany
Phone +49 681 37 20 271-1, Fax +49 681 37 20 271-0
Email: info@svh-verlag.de

Printed in the U.S.A.
Printed in the U.K. by (see last page)
ISBN: 978-3-8381-1203-9

Copyright © 2009 by the author and Südwestdeutscher Verlag für Hochschulschriften GmbH & Co. KG and licensors
All rights reserved. Saarbrücken 2009

Abstract

Image guided orthopedic intervention has seen rapid development in the past two decades. In many applications, the intraoperative use of medical imaging data has increased the safety and robustness of the surgical outcome. However it has also increased the applied radiation dose. Navigation systems were introduced in order to reduce the invasiveness of such procedures, while increasing the accuracy and safety of the procedures. The clinical procedures are often complex. Newly introduced systems often add more complexity and are not smoothly integrated into the clinical workflow. This thesis introduces two new concepts for computer aided surgery. Based on these concepts, it proposes innovative solutions satisfying the application specific requirements of the exemplary application for computer assisted spine surgery.

The first concept is based on a head mounted display for in-situ visualization. Initial clinical tests have shown that standard visualization methods based on volume and simple slice rendering are not sufficient for successfully performing surgical tasks. Therefore, a novel and promising alternative for in-situ guidance was designed, developed and evaluated, comprising a hybrid combination of standard slice-based visualization (commonly used during navigated procedures) with in-situ visualization. The second system is based on a mobile C-arm extended by a rigidly attached video camera originally proposed by Navab et al. [168]. The basic system enables image overlay of video and X-ray image without online calibration or registration. The newly designed and implemented extensions of this system facilitate guided instrumentation and a smooth integration into the surgical workflow.

During the technical evaluation and preclinical phantom and cadaver studies, both newly introduced concepts proved to offer promising support during image guided spine interventions. In addition to the traditional assessment of image guided surgery systems, a methodology is proposed for a reference-based assessment and a comparison between state-of-the-art, clinically used procedures and procedures based on the newly proposed systems. This methodology is based on the analysis of the clinical workflow, the design of simulated procedures, and their structured analysis. This model was applied to compare the newly developed camera augmented mobile C-arm system with the clinically applied fluoro CT guidance for vertebroplasty interventions.

Keywords:
Image-guided Surgery, Computer Assisted Surgery, Medical Augmented Reality, Workflow Based Assessment

Acknowledgments

First of all, I would like to thank my PhD adviser Nassir Navab a lot for the great opportunity to work in his research group for many years, making my dissertation possible, and for his always motivating and creative ideas, advice, guidance, and support during the last four and a half years. I also owe many thanks to Pierre Jannin who gave me great inspiration from his work and fruitful discussions about the assessment process for image guided interventions. Many thanks also to Ekkehard Euler who was very motivating for my subject on new concepts for orthopedic surgery and guided me during the last years through the medical application domain. Many thanks also to him for volunteering in many experiments and their evaluation. Thanks also to Bernd Bruegge who was more than just a chairman for my thesis. I would like to thanks Martin Horn and Martina Hilla for lot of support in organizational and administrative things. I also owe a great deal to Marco Feuerstein, Oliver Kutter, and Nicolas Padoy not only for proofreading my thesis, but also providing me together with Tobias Sielhorst lot of good advices, fruitful discussion and conduction of joint projects resulting in publications within the image guided surgery and medical augmented reality group at CAMP. It was my great pleasure to work with them during the last years. I would like to thank them as well as my colleagues and students Hauke Heibel, Selim Benhimane, Stefan Wiesner, Tassilo Klein, Tobias Reichl, Christoph Bichlmeier, Julian Much, Thomas Weich, Philipp Dressel, Lejing Wang, Philipp Stefan, who all assisted me greatly throughout my thesis and contributed to many joint publications. A special thanks goes to the CAMP workflow group Ahmad Ahmadi, Tobias Blum, and Nicolas Padoy for discussions and acquisition of the workflow for the vertebroplasty and simulated procedures. Furthermore, many thanks go to the rest of the CAMP team, namely Martin Groher, Ben Glocker, Christian Wachinger, Andreas Keil, Axel Martinez-Moeller, Martin Bauer, Stefan Hinterstoisser, Martin Horn, Moritz Blume, Pierre Georgel, Wolfgang Wein, Darko Zikic, Tobias Lasser, Ruxandra Micu, and many more, for making it possible to work in the most collaborative and pleasant environment including the frequent soccer matches.

I would also like to thank a lot Sandro M. Heining who was far more than a medical collaboration partner. He was very patient in introducing me to the everyday life of a trauma surgeon, helping me to develop many ideas, and for his advice and many fruitful discussions. I would like to thank him for his consultancy and joint conduction of experiments using the camera augmented mobile C-arm system and the head mounted display based augmented reality system as well as his colleagues Christian Riquarts and Ben Ockert.

I would like to thank Rainer Graumann from Siemens Medical SP for the support, fruitful discussions and many ideas for the camera augmented mobile C-arm system. Also

Frank Sauer and Ali Khamene from Siemens Corporate Research I owe great thanks for the design and development of the RAMP system as well as discussion about the extension of the concept for its usage in trauma surgery applications. Furthermore, many thanks go to Mark Schneberger, former ART GmbH for his support on the optical tracking system.

I was actively involved in a research project during the past four years that is not part of this thesis, but resulted in many publications. Therefore, I would like to thank especially Thomas Wendler for great support and many valuable discussions on various topics. Furthermore, I would like to thank Sibylle Ziegler for her advice in this project. Many thanks go also to further external collaboration partners Hubertus Feussner, Armin Schneider, and Peter Kneschaurek within other projects.

Finally, I owe a lot of thanks to my wife Stanka and my parents for their patience and great support during my thesis.

Contents

Acknowledgements   5

1 Image Guided Surgery   11
    1.1 Brief History of Image Guided Surgery 11
    1.2 Components of Image Guided Surgery Systems 15
       1.2.1 Medical Imaging 15
          1.2.1.1 X-ray 15
          1.2.1.2 Computed Tomography (CT) 17
          1.2.1.3 Magnetic Resonance Imaging (MRI) 17
          1.2.1.4 Ultrasonography (US) 18
          1.2.1.5 Single Photon Emission Computed Tomography (SPECT) and Position Emission Tomography (PET) 19
          1.2.1.6 Video Images (Microscopes, Endoscopic and Laparoscopic Imaging) 20
          1.2.1.7 Further Trends in Imaging Technologies 20
       1.2.2 Medical Signals and Models 22
       1.2.3 Tracking/Localization Systems 22
          1.2.3.1 Optical Infrared Tracking Systems 22
          1.2.3.2 Electromagnetic Tracking Systems 24
          1.2.3.3 Hybrid Tracking 25
       1.2.4 Human Computer Interaction and Data Representation 26
       1.2.5 Image Processing and Segmentation 27
       1.2.6 Registration 28
    1.3 Surgical Workflow Analysis 29
    1.4 Validation, Verification and Evaluation 31
       1.4.1 Related Work in Assessment of Medical Image Processing Methods   31
       1.4.2 Related Work in the Assessment of Image Guided Surgery Systems   32

Contents

2 Towards Advanced Visualization and Guidance   **35**
2.1 Towards Complex Image Guided Surgery Systems 35
2.2 Towards Full Integration of Patient and Procedure Specific Data 38
2.3 Towards Minimally Invasive Procedures in Orthopedic Surgery 40

3 Medical Application Domain   **43**
3.1 The Spine 43
    3.1.1 Spine Anatomy 43
    3.1.2 Access Trajectories to the Vertebrae 45
3.2 Spine Interventions 46
    3.2.1 Ventral Approach 46
    3.2.2 Dorsal Approach - Pedicle Screw Placements 47
    3.2.3 Dorsal Approach - Vertebroplasty 47
3.3 Computer Assisted Spine Interventions 48
    3.3.1 History of Computer Assisted Spinal Interventions 50
        3.3.1.1 Preoperative CT Navigation with External Tracking . . . 51
    3.3.2 2D C-arm/Fluoroscopy Guidance 53
    3.3.3 Three Dimensional Recoconstructed C-arm Guidance 53
        3.3.3.1 Discussion of Different Approaches for Navigated Spine Surgery 54

4 Two Novel Approaches to Image Guided Surgery   **55**
4.1 Hybrid Augmented Reality Navigation Interface 55
    4.1.1 Related Work in Head Mounted Display Based Augmented Reality 55
    4.1.2 System Components 56
        4.1.2.1 Hardware Setup 57
    4.1.3 Phantom Design and Clinical Integration 58
    4.1.4 Visualization Modes 61
        4.1.4.1 Standard Slice Based Navigation 61
        4.1.4.2 Augmented Reality Visualization Modes 61
        4.1.4.3 Hybrid Navigation Interface 64
    4.1.5 System Extensions to Enhance Depth Perception 64
4.2 Camera Augmented Mobile C-Arm (CamC) 66
    4.2.1 Related Work 66
    4.2.2 System Overview 67
        4.2.2.1 System Components 67
        4.2.2.2 System Calibration 68
        4.2.2.3 Implementation of System Calibration 71
        4.2.2.4 User Interface for Visualization and Navigation 73
    4.2.3 Clinical Applications 74
        4.2.3.1 Intraoperative Down-the-Beam Applications 74
        4.2.3.2 Alternative Clinical Applications 77
    4.2.4 System Extension for Enabling Depth Control 78
        4.2.4.1 System Setup 79
        4.2.4.2 Navigation and Surgical Workflow 82

		4.2.4.3	Preclinical Experiments with the Two Camera Solution	84
	4.2.5	\multicolumn{2}{l}{System Extension for Visual Servoing}	85
		4.2.5.1	System Configuration for Visual Servoing	87
		4.2.5.2	C-arm Kinematics	88
		4.2.5.3	Mathematical Problem Statement	88
		4.2.5.4	Two Dimensional Visual Servoing Algorithm	89
		4.2.5.5	Three Dimensional Visual Servoing Algorithm	91
		4.2.5.6	Evaluation of the Visual Servoing Algorithms	91
	4.2.6	\multicolumn{2}{l}{System Extension for X-ray Image Stitching}	92
		4.2.6.1	Method for X-ray Stitching:	94
		4.2.6.2	Parallax Effect	96
		4.2.6.3	Frontal Parallel Setup	97
		4.2.6.4	Implementation	97
		4.2.6.5	Experiments and Results	97

5 Assessment of Image Guided Surgery Systems — 101

5.1 Conventional Assessment of the Hybrid Augmented Reality Navigation Interface — 101

- 5.1.1 Technical Accuracy Evaluation — 101
  - 5.1.1.1 Single Camera Tracking Accuracy — 101
  - 5.1.1.2 Registration Accuracy — 102
  - 5.1.1.3 Instrument Tracking Accuracy — 103
  - 5.1.1.4 Synchronization Between Video Images and Tracking Data — 103
  - 5.1.1.5 Latency of the System — 103
- 5.1.2 Preclinical Evaluation — 104
  - 5.1.2.1 Evaluation of Depth Perception — 104
  - 5.1.2.2 Cadaver Study for Intramedullary Nail Locking — 104
  - 5.1.2.3 New Visualization Concepts and the Hybrid Interface — 105

5.2 Conventional Assessment of the Camera Augmented Mobile C-arm System — 111

- 5.2.1 Technical Accuracy Evaluation — 111
- 5.2.2 Preclinical Evaluation — 114
  - 5.2.2.1 Phantom and Cadaver Studies for Interlocking of Intramedullary Nails — 115
  - 5.2.2.2 Phantom Studies for Pedicle Approach - Vertebroplasty — 116
  - 5.2.2.3 Cadaver Studies for Pedicle Approach - Screw Placement — 116

5.3 Reference Based Assessment — 119

- 5.3.1 Workflow Analysis of the Clinical CT Fluoro Vertebroplasty Procedure — 120
- 5.3.2 Surgical Model of the Clinical CT Fluoro Vertebroplasty Procedure — 121
- 5.3.3 Design of a Simulated Surgical Procedure for Workflow Based Assessment in Vertebroplasty — 122
- 5.3.4 Workflow Analysis of Simulated Vertebroplasty Procedure using Fluoro CT and the Camera Augmented Mobile C-arm System — 122
- 5.3.5 Discussion of the Analysis of the Simulated Procedure — 125

Contents

6 Discussion and Conclusion   **127**
    6.1 Discussion 127
         6.1.1 Towards the Creation of System Models 128
         6.1.2 Towards the Integration of Surgical Models and Online Phase Detection in the Clinical Workflow 132
         6.1.3 Towards Standardized Preclinical Assessment of Image Guided Surgery Systems 133
    6.2 Conclusion 134

A Glossary   **137**

B Authored and Co-Authored Publications   **139**

References   **145**

CHAPTER 1

Image Guided Surgery

> The beginning of knowledge is
> the discovery of something we do not understand.
>
> *Frank Herbert (1920-1986)*

1.1 Brief History of Image Guided Surgery

Intraoperative navigation has evolved over the past decades in various fields of therapy. On the one hand there was the development of guided and assisted procedures, on the other hand the rapid development of medical imaging technologies and the diversification in the physical imaging properties, improvement in quality, resolution and reduction of acquisition time.

One of the first guided procedures in neurosurgery was reported by Dittmar in 1873, who used a guided probe to insert a blade into the medulla during an animal study [73]. This early neurosurgical guidance system did not incorporate any reference coordinate system that describes points and objects in three-dimensional space that is commonly used in today's navigation solutions. One of the first approaches for the stereotactic guidance, i.e. the relation of objects in Cartesian coordinates, was again in the domain of neurosurgery in the early 20th century by Horsley and Clarke(cf. figure 1.1) [67, 68, 74, 98]. They describe an apparatus to hold an electrode and guide it to a predefined location in three dimensions. That early system was only applied within animal studies. Only thirty years later, the combination with intraoperative X-ray imaging enabled the stereotactic guidance for clinical cases on humans by Spiegel and Wycis (cf. figure 1.2) [68, 222]. Current navigation suits are based on a very similar concept of attaching a reference base to the patient and either acquiring the imaging data within this reference frame or register the data to this reference frame.

One reason for the rapid development of image guided surgery in the last century was

Image Guided Surgery

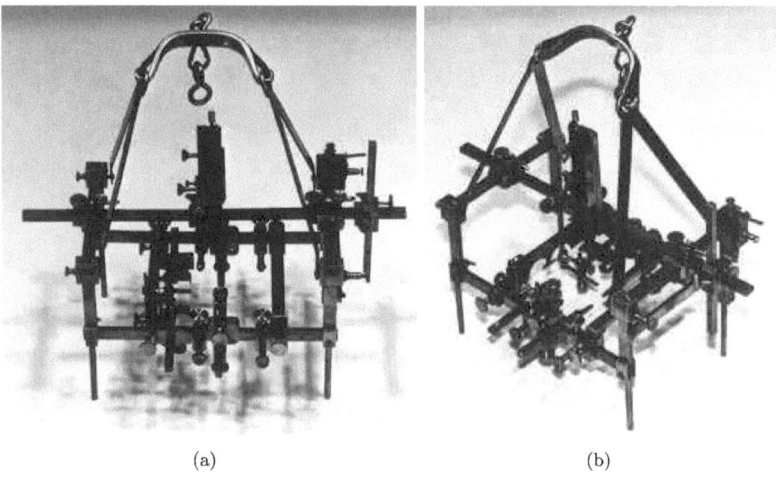

(a) (b)

Figure 1.1: The second Horsley-Clarke Stereotactic Instrument [98], constructed for Dr. Ernest Sachs in 1908 in London. Images courtesy of the Archives of the American Association of Neurological Surgeons.

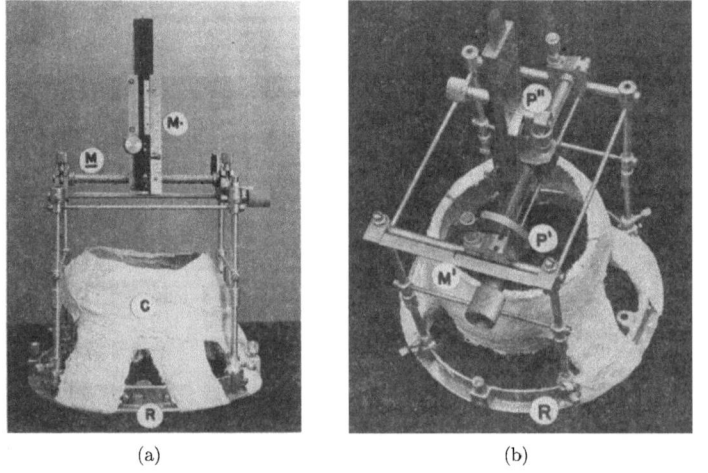

(a) (b)

Figure 1.2: Stereotaxic apparatus for operations on the human brain. From [222]. Reprinted with permission from AAAS.

1.1 Brief History of Image Guided Surgery

the invention of various medical imaging technologies. The development of endoscopic and laparoscopic techniques during the 19th century moved from direct vision to indirect vision onto the operation situs [19, 130, 137]. However, the physical properties of these endoscopic/laparoscopic imaging technologies were still based on the same principles as the vision of the human eye. The early apparatus were an extension of the human eye to look inside the patient's body through natural openings and/or small incisions. The advent of modern imaging technology and thus also image guided surgery was in 1895 with the invention of X-ray images by Konrad Röntgen in Würzburg, Germany [45]. A few months later the first clinical operation, based on this newly developed X-ray technology, was performed. In Birmingham, UK a needle was identified in the hand of a woman and removed with the help of a X-ray image in early 1896 [251]. The invention of X-ray imaging dating back to 1895 is nowadays still present in many everyday clinical routines. However, they are nowadays used in more sophisticated ways. The modern devices are capable of digital image acquisition, image enhancement, image processing and three-dimensional reconstruction. Also contrast enhanced acquisition and digitally subtracted radiographs contributed to the various application domains of X-ray technology. Especially the computed tomography (CT) that is based on X-ray imaging is a standard device for diagnostics and a traditional source of information for image guided surgery, especially in trauma and orthopedics surgery, where bony structures are the major focus. Other imaging devices like magnetic resonance imaging, ultrasound imaging, and molecular imaging techniques contribute to a more detailed and complete information for diagnosis, optimal treatment planning, optimized localization and categorization of suspicious regions.

Along with the development of imaging technologies there was the development of methods and apparatus for visualization and guidance. Most of the computer assisted surgery systems that are capable of navigation were developed in the past two decades with the wide availability and usability of computational processors[1], display devices and three-dimensional datasets. One early system for advanced visualization in image guided surgery, that is up to my knowledge the first method for in-situ visualization of imaging data was proposed by Steinhaus [224]. He presented in 1938 a visionary system that visualized the acquired X-rays directly on the operation situs. His construction placed an X-ray tube, a fluorescence plate, and a guidance construction such, that it was possible to guide an instrument to the desired target region (cf. figure 1.3). There was no report about a clinical application of the published technical system setup. Despite a few early and experimental systems, medical navigation systems were developed in the recent two decades.

Surveys, history, and various exemplary system setups and clinical applications for image guided surgery systems are summarized in several review papers [67, 183, 184, 185, 263], collection [131], special issue [245], and a textbook [184]. All of them describe the imaging technology as core and key component for the guidance systems. To fully enable a guidance system based on these images a spatial localization system and a technique to represent the information to the user are required as well as methods and algorithms for registration, calibration, segmentation, planning and visualization. The basic components

---

[1] first personal computer, IBM model 5150, was released in 1981

Image Guided Surgery

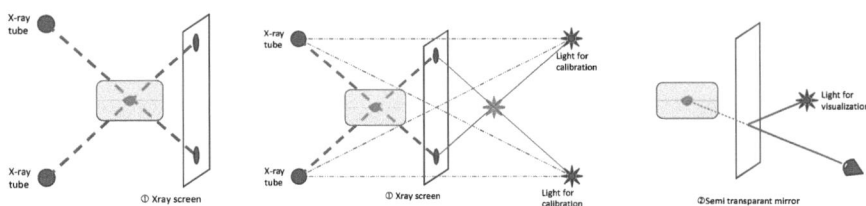

Figure 1.3: Calibration (left and middle) and in-situ visualization concept proposed by Steinhaus [224] in 1938. Image courtesy of Tobias Sielhorst [214].

of guidance systems will be discussed in more detail in the next section.

1.2 Components of Image Guided Surgery Systems

In this section the components and algorithms that are essential for image guided surgery systems are briefly introduced. First the components, i.e. medical imaging, models, localization systems, and human computer interfaces will be introduced, followed by the basic principles of registration and segmentation algorithms.

There is a huge diversity of proposed computer assisted surgery systems that were published and/or integrated into the surgery room in the past decades. The proposed systems cover the entire medical application domain based on diverse technology.

Surveys of image guided interventions identify the major components of computer assisted surgery systems to be imaging data, real time tracking systems (localization systems), data representation technologies, registration, planning, segmentation and interaction interfaces [67, 183, 185, 263]. Furthermore, monitoring, documentation, follow-up, workflow, and validation were recently added to the list of components.

1.2.1 Medical Imaging

In the traditional approach to image guided surgery the underlying information are medical image data. This is often the major source of information that is used for tailored, patient specific surgery, since it can provide both, anatomical and functional information. However, recent work in the research community proposed to include multiple other patient specific data as well as models of surgery and clinical cases into the navigation solution and especially into the selection of the right data representation [107, 169]. Standard protocols and data storage for patient specific data are available with the DICOM standard[2], that is currently extended to include patient specific therapy data within interventions in the DICOM24 workgroup, DICOM for surgery for standardized documentation of the treatment using image guided surgery systems [132]. Various medical imaging technologies based on different physical properties and setups customized towards different clinical requirements are available [90, 251, 260]. Some systems like X-ray, computed tomography, magnetic resonance imaging, ultrasound, positron emission tomography and single photon emission computed tomography (see the following subsections) are established, but research and development of new acquisition techniques is still an issue, especially in the domain of molecular imaging [261]. The increasing role of computers is mentioned with its possibility to converge diagnosis and therapy as well as the generation, processing, and fusion of all available information [261]. In this subsection of medical imaging only the very basic principles of the selected imaging technologies are introduced. References are provided for detailed information on the physical properties and medical applications of each introduced imaging system.

1.2.1.1 X-ray

The basic physical principle of X-ray is that X-ray photons are generated in a tube, sent through the human body and measured on a photon detector (cf. figure 4.11). The

---

[2]For the recent standard and announcements see http://medical.nema.org/

Image Guided Surgery

X-ray source and the detector are placed on the opposite side of the anatomy/object that is imaged. The measured activity of the detector shows the emitted value at the source minus the sum of the X-ray attenuation within the tissue that is traversed by the ray. Often similar models for the description of the X-ray geometry are applied as for optical cameras (cf. figure 4.10) commonly used in computer vision [83, 243, 266]. The relationship between a three dimensional object point and a two dimensional image point is represented by $x = PX$ with $P \in \mathbb{R}^{3\times 4}$ being the projection matrix, $X \in \mathbb{P}^3$ the object point in 3D and $x \in \mathbb{P}^2$ its corresponding point in the image in projective space [210]. The major differences are that X-ray images are not surface images, but projective images, the direction of the rays goes from the source to the detector, and the source and detector are decoupled and not in the same housing.

Classical application domains for X-ray imaging are to analyze bony structures, since bones have a high X-ray attenuation compared to other tissue. The digitalization of images in combination with contrast agents introduced digitally subtracted radiographs to visualize vessel structures. In intervention rooms there exist stationary (angiography) and mobile (C-arm) solutions. They are used during the intervention for real time fluoroscopic image feedback e.g. in applications for catheter placement, instrument guidance, or three dimensional reconstructions. Mobile C-arms are commonly used as a supporting tool during orthopedic and trauma surgeries. Its advantages are the real time image acquisition, its flexible usage, and its wide availability in the operating room. Its disadvantages are radiation hygienic reasons and that a standard X-ray image can only provide two dimensional projective images. Real time three dimensional or two dimensional tomographic reconstructed images are not available with standard X-ray imaging devices and C-arms.

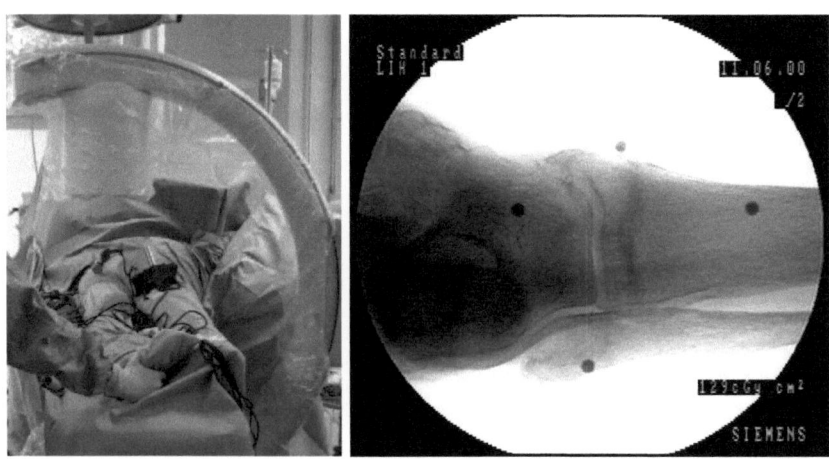

(a) Mobile C-arm device. (b) X-ray image of a foot.

Figure 1.4: Mobile C-arm used during orthopedic surgery and an exemplary X-ray image generated by the device.

1.2 Components of Image Guided Surgery Systems

1.2.1.2 Computed Tomography (CT)

Based on similar physical attenuation properties than two dimensional projective X-ray images CT fluoro slices and three dimensional CT datasets are generated. The X-ray source and detector (array) are rotated around the anatomy/object in order acquire the X-ray attenuation profiles at poses with a minimum of 180 degree rotation around the anatomy/object. Standard closed CT scanners (cf. figure 1.5(a)) perform rotations of source and detector around 360 degrees with multiple spins per second[3] while the bed and patinet are translated through the gantry. The detector consists of several scan rows that simultaneously scan the patient (for multislice scanners that are currently available up to 128 slices). Intraoperative C-arms and O-arm[4] systems that are capable of three dimensional reconstruction use so called cone beam reconstructions [54]. The acquired attenuation is not measured by a linear array of detectors, but by a two dimensional array, which results in two dimensional projective X-ray image. Algebraic or Fourier methods are used to reconstruct the volume. CT images are used in diagnostics for trauma and orthopedic surgery, tumor detection (screening) and detection of abnormalities as well as in therapy for image guidance interventions. Recent scanners (e.g. the Siemens SOMATOM Sensation 64-slice configuration) have a high quality and can also distinguish between different soft tissue.

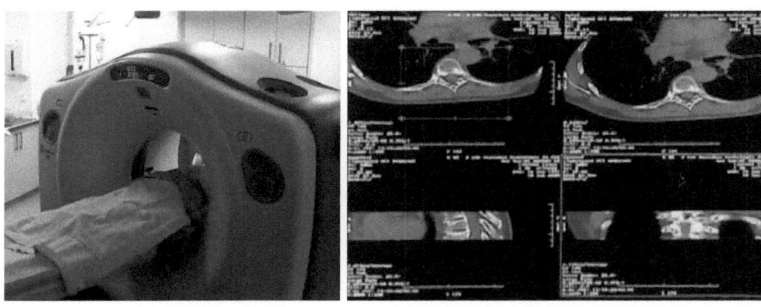

(a) 64 slice CT scanner. (b) Spiral CT 3D dataset.

Figure 1.5: CT scanner (Siemens SOMATOM Sensation 64-slice configuration), here used for vertebroplasty procedure.

1.2.1.3 Magnetic Resonance Imaging (MRI)

A powerful imaging technology for soft tissue and tumor classification, as well as for functional imaging data is magnetic resonance imaging. The technique is based on the excitement of nucleis within a strong magnetic field. This applied strong magnetic field aligns hydrogen atoms in the body. An alternating magnetic field is used to manipulate the

---
[3]The Siemens SOMATOM Sensation performs currently three spins per second.
[4]http://www.medtronicnavigation.com/procedures/intraoperative/o-arm.jsp

Image Guided Surgery

orientation of the nucleis/hydrogen atoms in the body along the magnetic field lines. They emit a weak radio signal which is amplified and measured by detectors. The alternating magnetic field manipulates the signal in order to acquire enough information to generate an image. The pulsing magnetic field brings a nuclei in a higher energy state and its relaxation and realignment emits energy that is measured. The realignment of nuclear spins with the magnetic field is termed longitudinal relaxation and the time required for a certain percentage of the nuclei to realign is termed T1 (for a T1 Tse MRI image of the spine cf. figure 1.6(b)), which is typically around one second for tissue. T2-weighted imaging (for a T2 Stir sequence cf. figure 1.6(a), cf. figure 1.6(c) for a T2 Tse sequence) relies upon local dephasing of spins following the application of a transverse energy pulse. This is typically smaller than 100 ms for tissue. For the generation of a two dimensional slice image of the measured T1 or T2 a Fourier approach is used in general. MRI has much higher soft tissue contrast than CT imaging and is used for diagnosis in neurological, musculoskeletal, cardiovascular, and oncological diseases. The physical property of strong magnetic fields and its long acquisition times when high image quality is required limits its usage mainly for diagnostic purposes. Some researchers propose its usage in form of open scanners in the operation room for neurosurgical applications [29, 225], prostate [123], and other oncological applications [43, 51]. They all designed environments and clinical procedures that are entirely compatible with strong magnetic fields, including the design of new devices, instrumentation, and all other equipment. The size of the scanner, the magnetic field, and long acquisition times are challenges for engineers and its clinical acceptance.

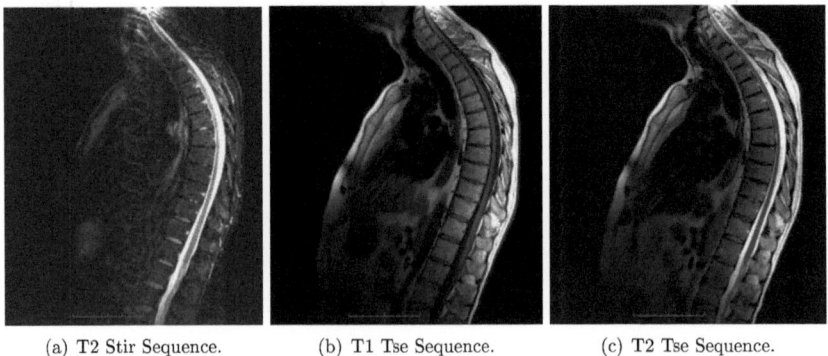

(a) T2 Stir Sequence.   (b) T1 Tse Sequence.   (c) T2 Tse Sequence.

Figure 1.6: Magnetic resonance image of the spine and spinal cord. Different sequences are shown in the sagittal plane.

1.2.1.4 Ultrasonography (US)

Ultrasonography is a powerful non invasive anatomical and functional imaging modality for diagnosis and therapy (cf. figure 1.7). It is a modality that requires images in real time

1.2 Components of Image Guided Surgery Systems

in two or three dimensions with high spatial resolution and without ionizing radiation. Furthermore, it can be used to create functional imaging data. Despite its limitation that is noise in the image, shadowing effects, and a low penetration, it provides a good imaging technology for image guided surgery. The basic principle of ultrasonography is the generation of sound waves, the measurement of their echo, and their interpretation. In a standard ultrasound device the sound wave is generated in a transducer element array within the ultrasound probe. The frequencies range between two and fifteen MHz. The received echoes are used for the image generation, in particular the direction of the echo, the amplitude of the echo and the temporal delay between the emission of the sound wave and the receiving echo. Ultrasonography is used for a wide range of applications in diagnostics and therapy. Higher frequency ultrasound (7-15MHz), and thus lower wavelength, is used to image structures close to the surface like muscles and neonatal brain and provides better axial and lateral resolution. Lower frequency ultrasound (2-7MHz), and thus higher wavelength, is used for deeper located structures like liver and kidney. There exist three dimensional ultrasound devices that generate a volume either using a transducer element matrix or by moving a transducer array. Its limitation are the physical nature of ultrasound waves in gas, thus a physical contact of the probe with the anatomy always needs to be established. There are miniature ultrasound probes available for laparoscopic, endoscopic, and intravascular applications.

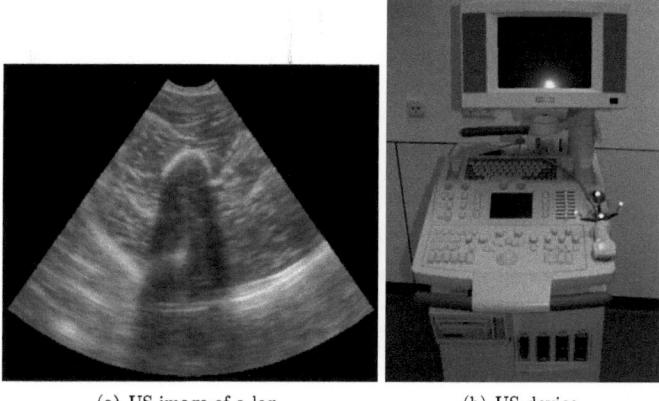

(a) US image of a leg.   (b) US device.

Figure 1.7: Ultrasound image of the Wachingersche leg with clear visible artifacts in the center of the image (shadowing effects) and an ultrasound device including the probe.

1.2.1.5 Single Photon Emission Computed Tomography (SPECT) and Position Emission Tomography (PET)

SPECT and PET are nuclear medicine imaging techniques. SPECT is using the detection of gamma rays, similar to the technique of gamma or anger cameras [5, 182], but

Image Guided Surgery

with a three dimensional reconstruction of the acquired information generating three dimensional datasets. Gamma cameras measure the projection of gamma radiation from a specific viewpoint, or more precise, they accumulate the gamma radiation that is emitted in the direction of the detector array. SPECT uses multiple of such gamma camera projections for a tomographic reconstruction of the measured activity in three dimensions. The measured activity is emitted by a radionucleid that is injected and accumulates at specific regions. Commonly used tracer are Technetium-99m (^{99m}Tc) for functional brain imaging and Indium-111 (^{111}In) for tumor scans. Its major application domain is in tumor imaging, but also imaging of infected regions. It is furthermore used for functional imaging of internal organs like brain and heart [257]. In contrast to SPECT, PET does not detect the direct emission of gamma rays, but it detects pairs of gamma rays on the so called line of response that are indirectly generated by a positron emitting radioisotope. Thus, the basic principle of the device is not a rotating gamma camera, but a ring of detector bins around the object [187, 257]. Radionuclides used in PET scanning are typically isotopes with short half lives such as carbon-11 ($\approx$20 min), nitrogen-13 ($\approx$10 min), oxygen-15 ($\approx$2 min), and Fluorine-18 ($\approx$110 min). Radioactive tracer isotopes, that are responsible for the emitting positron and thus the gamma rays are injected and accumulated in the tissue of interest. The molecule used for the metabolic process is most commonly fluorodeoxyglucose (FDG).

1.2.1.6 Video Images (Microscopes, Endoscopic and Laparoscopic Imaging)

The increased motivation for minimally invasive procedures developed instruments for indirect vision into the region of interest either by rigid (e.g. laparoscope or arthroscope) or flexible (e.g. bronchoscope, gastroscope, or colonoscope) instruments. The general aim is less trauma of the patient enabled by an entry of the optical instrument through small incisions (ports) or natural body openings (e.g. bronchoscope introduced trough nose and trachea into the airways). In general instruments are composed of a light source, an optic, a video camera at the proximal end, and a working channel for the insertion of instruments e.g. biopsy needles. The size of the instruments range from 0.1 to 2 cm in diameter and from 10 cm to over 1 m in length, depending on the particular application [32]. The devices are used for diagnosis and therapy. They are well established in many disciplines of surgery. Several systems were proposed recently using enhanced endoscope systems for soft tissue navigation [15].

1.2.1.7 Further Trends in Imaging Technologies

Despite the commonly used and above introduced imaging technologies, there are several alternative modalities that will provide additional information, especially functional information about patients' tissue properties. One example that enables access to new information is molecular imaging, the minimally invasive in vivo sensing, depiction, and characterization of spatially localized biologic processes at the cellular and molecular level [36]. Molecular imaging devices are currently developed along with the development of novel molecular agents, that attach with a high level of specificity to genes, proteins, or other molecular targets and can be imaged with various techniques [212].

1.2 Components of Image Guided Surgery Systems

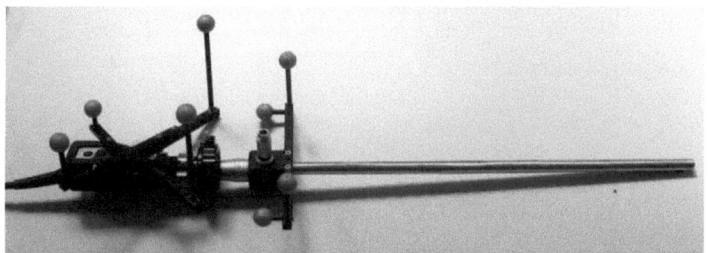

Figure 1.8: A laparoscope with a oblique viewing 30 degree optic. The laparoscope is extended by tracking targets to enable soft tissue navigation as proposed by Feuerstein et al. [55].

Other exemplary new technology for functional imaging, are nuclear probes, which provide an imaging modality with the flexibility for intraoperative usage [93]. Probes or cameras detecting beta or gamma radiation can be used hand-held in an operation suite in comparison to diagnostic functional imaging devices like SPECT or PET. The probes simply provide a one dimensional signal of measured activity and cameras two dimensional projections of the radioactive distribution in space [18]. In our group, we extended standard nuclear (beta and gamma) probes by a spatial localization system (cf. section 1.2.3) to extend the one dimensional signal of the probe to generate two dimensional surfaces or reconstruct three dimensional images [170]. For beta radiation, which has the property that it does not penetrate tissue more than two millimeters, we create color encoded surface maps that show the activity [256]. The gamma radiation penetrates the tissue and can thus be measured also if it is located deep inside the situs. The combination of such a gamma probe with a localization system enables the reconstruction of a three dimensional volume [255]. In addition we proposed an integration of a gamma probe with an ultrasound probe for combined anatomical and functional guided nodule resection enabled by real time fusion of all information within the operating room [254].

A further promising and emerging technology of molecular imaging is optical imaging. The basic technique of optical and near infrared imaging is similar to X-ray imaging. A source excites the waves through the patient anatomy and a detector measures the quantity that penetrates the tissue. Optical tomography is an extension with a source exciting the detector from many different directions. One clinical example is the tomographic laser mammography. Additional emerging imaging technologies that have not yet found their clinical applications, but show promising results are thermography, electrocardiography and electroencephalography, magnetocardiography and magnetoencephalography, terahertz imaging, tissue impedance imaging, and electron-spin resonance imaging. This is just a selection of novel imaging technologies [261].

Image Guided Surgery

1.2.2 Medical Signals and Models

Other than medical imaging data there are various patient specific data like electroencephalography (EEG) that can contribute to diagnostic and therapy decisions during computer assisted treatments. So far few researchers paid attention to all the available patient data in the intervention room. Jannin et al. incorporate all patient specific data like sex, age into their model of the surgery [107]. Padoy et al. incorporate online detected biosignals in order to analyze and predict the current workflow phase during an intervention [180].

To complete the patient specific data, explicit knowledge of the anatomy, physiology, and surgical case are components of an image guided surgery system. There is extensive work in the generation of atlas data, especially for neurosurgical applications [233]. Patient specific images can be registered to atlas data and thus allow the classification of specific regions. Besides inter subject models, models of surgeries are of clinical relevance. In general this knowledge is assumed to be implicit within the physician's mind. In section 1.3 novel attempts of workflow and surgical models, as well as its applications are discussed in details.

1.2.3 Tracking/Localization Systems

Tracking systems are used to spatially localize an object with respect to another object or a reference coordinate system. In general six degree-of-freedom pose data, which are composed of three degrees of freedom for translation and three degrees of freedom for rotation, are reported by such systems. There are various technologies available, e.g. based on cameras, electromagnetic fields, inertial sensors, sound waves, or mechanic links [28, 195, 253]. In image guided surgery spatial localization systems can also be imaging devices like fluoroscopy or ultrasound in combination with an appropriate segmentation and classification algorithm to detect the objects of interest in the images. A catheter can be tracked within fluoroscopic or ultrasonic images and guided with this information towards the planned target location. The requirements for tracking systems to be used in image guided surgery are accuracy, reliability and clinical usability. Optical and electromagnetic tracking system are the most commonly used systems despite of medical imaging data [24, 27]. The technology of optical and electromagnetic tracking are addressed in the next two subsections 1.2.3.1 and 1.2.3.2 along with their advantages and limitations. Hybrid tracking, as a combination of two tracking systems to overcome the shortcomings of each individual system is introduced in section 1.2.3.3, with a focus on the combination of optical and electromagnetic tracking.

1.2.3.1 Optical Infrared Tracking Systems

Optical tracking systems used in image guided surgery are in general composed of two or more cameras. The basic idea is to detect the same feature simultaneously within two or more cameras and reconstruct this feature in three dimensions using a known camera geometry and the relation between the cameras. The estimation of the camera models and their relation are well known techniques in computer vision [53, 83]. In order to detect features in the camera images with a high confidence level, infrared technology is used i.e. the cameras are equipped with an infrared filter to image only the infrared spectrum of the light. There exist passive and active infrared tracking solutions. Active systems use infrared emitting diodes. Passive systems use infrared retroreflective material and a ring of infrared flashes mounted around the cameras. One single feature point allows localizing

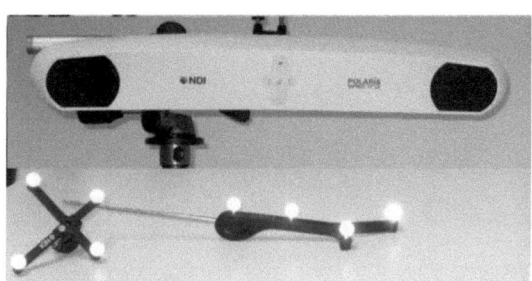
(a) Tracking cameras and exemplary tracking targets.

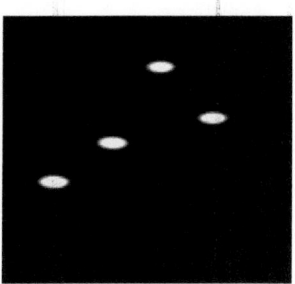
(b) Image of a target in the infrared camera.

Figure 1.9: An exemplary optical infrared tracking system to localize targets with six degrees of freedom.

it in three dimensions using a minimum of two cameras with a known camera model and a known correspondence between the features in the two images. A known three dimensional geometric configuration of a minimum of three features allows the estimation of the position and the orientation of the arrangement using the constraints that they are not on one line and that they describe an asymmetric pattern. These arrangements are often called targets or rigid bodies and are rigidly attached to instruments and patient anatomy (cf. figure 1.10).

Commonly used systems are the Optotrak™ and Polaris™ (Northern Digital Inc., Ontario, Canada). Their accuracy was evaluated together with the FlashPoint™ (Image Guided Technologies, Inc., Boulder, Colorado) system [42, 115]. The Optotrak system shows the highest reliability, especially in terms of fast target movements, and the accuracy, especially the rotational accuracy, was significantly higher compared to the other systems [42]. Its only disadvantages are the high price and the bigger size compared to the Polaris™ and Flashpoint™ systems.

For a very limited working volume the Veicra™ (Northern Digital Inc., Ontario, Canada) was recently introduced with a smaller baseline of the cameras and thus a smaller working volume with high accuracy.

An alternative to the rigid arrangement of the tracking cameras is a system based on the ARTtrack™ cameras (A.R.T. Advanced Realtime Tracking GmbH, Weilheim, Germany) since it allows a flexible arrangement of up to sixteen cameras. This however introduces additional challenges to ensure the accuracy within the tracking volume. The accuracy depends to a large extend on the arrangement of the cameras and the visibility of the markers in the individual cameras. The uncertainty of a single feature/marker, its con-

Image Guided Surgery

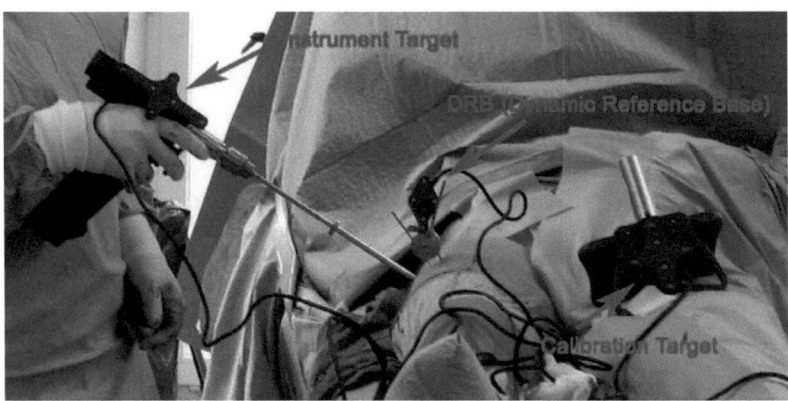

Figure 1.10: On the left hand side a surgical drill is extended by a six degree of freedom optical tracking target. A reference marker target (DRB) is screwed into the femur of the patient. On the right hand side there is a calibration target for the calibration of the drill. The image shows an navigated surgery at Klinikum Innenstadt by Prof. E. Euler and Dr. S. M. Heining using the Medivision navigation system.

tribution to the accuracy in the three dimensional estimation of a single feature/marker, and its propagation towards the target region have to be integrated to ensure the reliability of such a system. Bauer et al. [13, 14] and Sielhorst et al. [215] showed the propagation of the error and the influence of transformations, marker fusion, and hidden markers to the uncertainty of the tracking result.

1.2.3.2 Electromagnetic Tracking Systems

Electromagnetic tracking (EMT) is widely used in medical applications [195] and is the only posibility to track flexible instruments without the usage of medical image data. One of its main advantages compared to other tracking systems is that there is no requirement for a direct line-of-sight, i.e. also sensors inside the patient without visual contact to the field generator can be localized. Electromagnetic tracking systems are based on the generation of electromagnetic fields to estimate the position and orientation of sensors [188]. A typical electromagnetic tracking system setup consists of an electromagnetic field transmitter or generator and one or more electromagnetic sensors. Within the transmitter, three orthogonal coils are used to generate a magnetic field by means of current induction. Similarly, the receiver also contains orthogonal miniaturized coils. Within a specified tracking volume (cf. figure 1.11(b)) current is induced into the coils of the sensor. Based on the strength of the induced current and a comparison between received and sent signal the position and orientation of the sensor relative to the transmitter is estimated and reported by the system. There exist two systems that are used within medical applications. The NDI Aurora® system (Northern Digital Inc., Ontario, Canada) and the

1.2 Components of Image Guided Surgery Systems

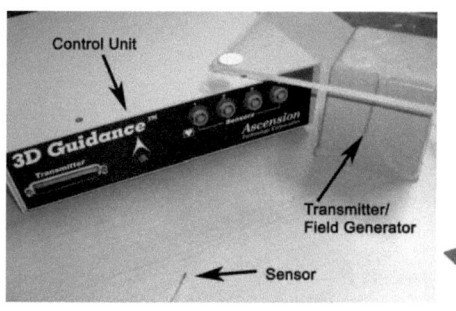
(a) Electromagnetic tracking system.

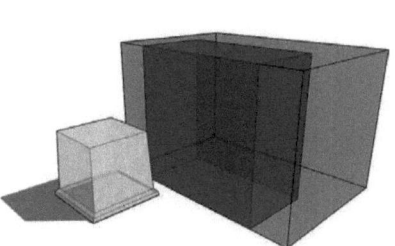
(b) Tracking volume.

Figure 1.11: The 3D Guidance™System (Ascension Technology Corporation) and its tracking volume as an example for an electromagnetic tracking system. The gray volume is for the sensor model 180, a large volume senser, the blue one for the sensor model 130, a small volume sensor.

3D Guidance™(Ascension Technology Corporation, Burlington, VT, USA). Despite their advantage that they do not require direct line-of-sight between the transmitter and sensor, their major limitations are the relatively small tracking volume and the perturbance of the generated electromagnetic field [27, 207]. Especially ferromagnetic material and inductive materials perturb the electromagnetic field. Detailed evaluation of currently existing systems, especially in the presence of ferromagnetic material, was performed by Hummel et al. [99, 100, 101]. There are several attempts to correct for perturbed electromagnetic measurements. Static field errors can be compensated by the acquisition of a ground truth and a function that maps the perturbed data to its real data [116, 139]. In our lab we implemented an error correction based on the acquisition of the ground truth data with a high accurate optical tracking system and hardy's multiquadric interpolation method [236]. Another research issue in the field of electromagnetic tracking is the detection of dynamic perturbance of the electromagnetic field by moving equipment, devices, and instruments in a close vicinity to the transmitter and/or sensor. Setups were proposed to detect a dynamically perturbed electromagnetic field using two rigidly attached sensors and measure their deviation over time [160, 161]. Recently, we proposed two methods for error correction in electromagnetic tracking without the explicit knowledge of the error model. The first method is based on a hybrid combination of an optical and an electromagnetic tracking system [56, 58]. The second method is based on a model of the motions, the configuration space of our instruments, assuming we can track the distal end of the instruments with a stable, high accurate tracking system, e.g. an optical tracking system [57].

1.2.3.3 Hybrid Tracking

Several attempts were proposed to combine two complementary tracking technologies in order to overcome their individual shortcomings. The first hybrid systems for medical applications were proposed by Birkfellner et al. [26, 27]. They propose the combination of external optical infrared tracking systems with electromagnetic tracking solutions. The same combination was proposed by Auer and Pinz [9] for head tracking within augmented reality applications. A slightly different hybrid approach was proposed by Mori et al. [159]. They extend a tracking algorithm based on image registration between real and virtual bronchoscopy images by an electromagnetic tracking system. Further hybrid solutions were proposed by Nakamoto et al. [162] and by Feuerstein et al. , within our group, [56, 57, 58] for opto-electromagnetic tracking within laparoscopic interventions with partly rigid and partly deformable instruments and devices.

1.2.4 Human Computer Interaction and Data Representation

Troccaz and Merloz recently identified that not much effort has so far made for an ideal human computer interface for computer assisted orthopedic surgery [241]. Their definition of an ideal interface is that it is omnipresent, but invisible. This was achieved over the past decades in many non medical domains, like cars and electronic devices, where computers are integrated, but their complexity is to a large extend hidden from the end user. The questions what information is required, in which form and during which distinct moments within an intervention requires formalisms and representations [109]. A complete analysis and implementation of this formalism will allow predictive and workflow driven user interfaces [169] that make full advantage of available technologies e.g. augmented reality systems [217, 237], which is the overlay of virtual data (here medical image data) onto the view of the physician.

One suitable model to classify the interaction between user and system in the presence of an augmented reality system is described in [49], but was later used to also describe interaction in general computer assisted surgery systems. The four major components in an augmented reality system are identified as object (O), person (P), adapter (A), and system (S). Objects and persons are always communicating with the system using adapters (cf. figure 1.2.4). The so called OP-a-S Model (Object, Person, adapter, System) was used to derive a methodology to explain why a surgeon had problems with the interpretation of specific navigation information [48]. An extension to this model is the categorization

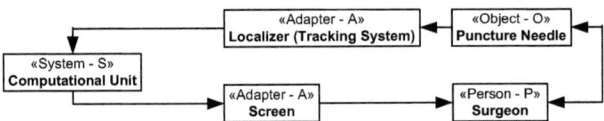

Figure 1.12: The object, person, adapter, system model (OP-a-S) showing the interaction of a computer assisted surgery system [48, 49].

of the adapters in input (e.g. keyboard or tracking system) and output (e.g. display) adapters [145]. A further refinement is their classification into indirect and direct adapter situations.

1.2 Components of Image Guided Surgery Systems

- Indirect input situation: $P \rightarrow A_{in} \rightarrow S$ e.g. the classical computer interaction using a mouse or a keyboard.

- Direct input situation: $P \rightarrow [R_{tool}, R_{object}] \rightarrow A_{in} \rightarrow S$ e.g. the spatial relationship between the tool and the surgical object is in a specific constellation.

- Indirect output situation: $S \rightarrow A_{out} \rightarrow P$ e.g. the classical data representation method on a screen.

- Direct output situation: $S \rightarrow A_{out} \rightarrow [R_{tool}, R_{object}] \rightarrow P$ e.g. the use of assitance arms or $S \rightarrow A_{out} \rightarrow R_{object} \rightarrow P$ e.g. the use of an in-situ visualization system.

A trend for data representation is the use of augmented reality to provide the information in-situ. A commonly accepted definition of augmented reality by Azuma is that it combines real and virtual data, interactively in real time and registered in three dimensions [10, 11]. In medicine several applications were proposed in the past [205, 214, 217]. Bajura et al. first proposed the usage of augmented reality technology based on a head mounted display (HMD) that visualizes the acquired ultrasound image of a pregnant woman's abdomen [12]. Especially the combination of the augmented reality in-situ visualization technology with existing imaging devices showed a promising integration into the clinical workflow. King et al. [117] proposed a system that extends an operating microscope and integrates the three dimensional imaging information into the operation situs for neurosurgery. Birkfellner and Figl et al. [25, 59] integrated the augmented reality technology into an existing head mounted operating microscope commonly used during maxillofacial surgery. Stetten and Chib [226] combined an ultrasound device with a half silvered mirror and a monitor in such an arrangement that by construction the acquired image is registered with the patient's anatomy. Navab et al. [168] extend a mobile C-arm by a video camera and a double mirror construction such that the video image is registered with the X-ray image by construction (cf. section 4.2).

Fuchs et al. [66] and Sauer at al. [202] report systems based on head mounted display technologies, just to name two further examples of in-situ visualization with the ultimate goal to provide an intuitive three dimensional user interface for representation of medical information within image guided surgery.

1.2.5 Image Processing and Segmentation

A classical domain in medical image computing and image guided interventions is the image processing, filtering, and segmentation of data [186, 174]. It is a fundamental contribution to image guided surgery used for classification, tracking, interpretation, and visualization of medical imaging data. There are various algorithms available starting from simple thresholding and region growing towards more complex algorithms and optimizations like graph cut algorithm [34] towards algorithms based on dynamic contours like snakes [113] or level set [178, 211].

1.2.6 Registration

Another classical domain in medical image computing and image guided interventions is registration, i.e. the alignment of datasets in a common coordinate frame [81, 144, 262]. Special focus in image guided interventions is the patient to modality registration, i.e. to align the medical imaging data within the physical coordinate system of the patient, which is often defined by a spatial localization system. There is a wide range of methods from standard point based rigid registration [8, 244], over surface [20, 265] and volume registration [118], towards non-rigid registration [84]. The errors within registration procedures have to be quantified and propagated in order to estimate its final influence on the provided navigation [61]. A methodology to validate image registration procedures was proposed in [104].

1.3 Surgical Workflow Analysis

The magnitude of available information and possibilities for treatment lead to a complex decision process for the optimal treatment delivery. The aim of workflow analysis and surgical models is to recover and model the surgical procedures, analyze and interpret them using ontologies, and the creation of case specific surgical models. This chapter will summarize the achievements in workflow analysis and surgical modeling that can be classified in online and offline procedures, preoperative and intraoperative procedures, manual and automatic approaches, as well as systems dedicated to study the surgical skills.

Surgical workflow analysis aims at modeling the process of events within an intervention. Burgert et al. [41] built a high level ontology to describe items, actions and their spatial and temporal relationship. The structured manual recording during an intervention is done with a custom developed software on a touchscreen device and stored in a database enabled by XML [172]. The visualization of the workflow was proposed as time-related representation, i.e. sequential and parallel order of actions, or as logic-oriented representation, i.e. the control flow of events [173].

Another group that is working on issues for structured reporting and documentation is the DICOM WG24 with the objective to create standards and modeling techniques for image guided surgery [132]. This was motivated by many complex system in the operating room that are unable to communicate due to missing standardized interfaces. They define goals and items for standards that will be the fundament of integrated and exchangeable solutions in the operating room of the future. This is enabled by the specification and design of a therapy imaging and model management system (TIMMS) proposed by Lemke et al. [133]. The ultimate goal will be to establish interchangeable objects in the operating room and communication between modules to enable the optimal patient outcome in image guided surgery, communication between the modules and the documentation of the procedures.

A different approach is the work by Jannin at al. [107, 108]. They define a surgery model based on the unified modeling language (UML) that manages all available multimodal information (e.g. patient information, anatomical and functional imaging data). They show the validity of their model with neurosurgical procedures. However, the defined model will be also valid for other interventional procedures. They divide a surgical procedure into several successive phases, each containing a set of imaging entities required to fulfill this step. In a study, neurosurgeons defined the required imaging data at specific steps of the procedure in advance and the use of this imaging entity was validated during the procedure [107]. This is done in order to support the surgical strategy for patient individual treatment, to improve the human computer interface of computer assisted surgical systems and to formalize explicit surgical knowledge and practice. The models are mainly generated preoperatively and validated intraoperative observing the actions and decisions of surgeons.

Within our group Ahmadi et al. [2] proposed a method for the creation of a model for surgery without an underlying structure by recording synchronized signals. The early system enables the recording and temporal synchronization of various signals during an

Image Guided Surgery

intervention. Additionall a custom developed software is used for simultaneous playback of surgeries with all the recorded information (e.g. video cameras, laparoscopic camera, and movement of surgical staff) [220]. Also low level signal processing was integrated into their approach to automatically extract information by classification of video images The method was further extended to obtain an accurate offline detection of surgical phases [179]. The incorporation of image processing methods and patterns during surgery was an initial step towards online phase detection [181]. This was refined and used for an online generation of surgical model based on hidden markov models [31]. Other groups are also performing low level signal and image processing to find patterns on-line within surgical procedures enabled by used (laparoscopic/endoscopic) or added (video) cameras in the operating room [141].

A different approach, with the aim at assessing the surgical skill and performance is proposed by various groups, also based in synchronized acquisition of data including video images [136, 151, 196, 197].

Within this thesis the recording and analysis of the workflow is used to assess different parameters for the evaluation of new image guided surgery solutions, by comparing the standard procedure with a surgical simulation. The tools developed within our group were used to record and label surgical actions in order to allow a comparison between the workflow steps to get a more detailed analysis than comparing only the duration and accuracy of the entire procedure.

1.4 Validation, Verification and Evaluation

There is a general need for validation, verification and evaluation of procedures in image guided surgery not only in medical product development with the regulations and norms (FDA 510k[5], CE 93/42/EWG[6]), but also within research prototypes. The assessment is often a tedious process. Its non rigorous design, conduction, and reporting is a major drawback and makes the results of experiments and studies not transparent. The standard approach to assessment in image guided surgery systems is to evaluate the technical parameters of the system (e.g. precision and accuracy), followed by simulated procedures within a laboratory setup with phantom, cadaver and in-vivo animal experiments towards patient trials in the operating room. For complex systems this is a long lifecycle and a time and money consuming process.

The terms verification, validation, and evaluation describe different parts of the assessment in an image guided surgery system. Verification is the process of analyzing the system if it was build according to the specified requirements. Validation is the analysis if the system fulfills the purpose it was designed for [102]. Evaluation is the analysis of the benefit of a system in various dimensions. Assessment is the process of gathering and analyzing specific information as part of an evaluation.

1.4.1 Related Work in Assessment of Medical Image Processing Methods

A methodology was proposed for standardized conduction and reporting of validation, verification and evaluation in medical image processing (e.g. medical image registration, segmentation) [104]. These assessments are crucial since image processing methods are always subsystems of complex setups for image guided surgery. Jannin et al. [104] claim that a standardized protocol of validation methodology and a standardized data set will be the key success to a valid and comparable assessment of image processing methods. They furthermore derive six evaluation layers from a method that was previously proposed to assess the efficacy of diagnostic imaging systems [65]. These six layers are:

1. technical capacity, i.e. the intrinsic technical parameters of the system

2. diagnostic accuracy, i.e. the system accuracy on relevant anatomical or pathological structures

3. diagnostic impact, i.e. improvement or change in diagnostic protocols

4. therapeutic impact, i.e. change in the decision for delivery of the treatment

5. patient outcome, i.e. the benefit of the patient health and individual quality of life

6. social impact, e.g. cost effectiveness and change in health care system and general quality of life

---
[5]Premarket Notification (PMN) that is required by the U.S. Food and Drug Administration at least 90 days in prior to market a medical device http://www.fda.gov/cdrh/510khome.html
[6]The European guidlines for medical device manufacterer.

Most of the proposed research systems and algorithms in literature are only evaluated on the first two of these layers that are performed in the lab and a simulated surgery. The transition of research prototypes into the operation room is often a major barrier for radical new solutions. The initial step is accessing the system parameters and technical accuracy, i.e. intrinsic parameters of an algorithm. The second layer is the evaluation of the accuracy of an algorithm or image processing procedure based on realistic data and a ground truth measurement method.

The general technical requirements for a transparent and comparable validation of different medical image processing methods include a standardization of validation methodology, design of validation data sets, and validation metrics. This is in general only possible in the same or similar application domains and with similar algorithms of image processing. It becomes even more complex with the assessment of a complete image guided surgery system.

1.4.2 Related Work in the Assessment of Image Guided Surgery Systems

The proposed concept for assessment in diagnostic imaging systems [65] and medical image processing methods [104] was also adopted for the assessment of systems for image guided intervention by Jannin and Korb [106, 121]. The layer concept was refined for image guided interventions. In most levels the impacts during a surgery are divided into indirect i.e. diagnostic values and direct i.e. therapeutic values. The refined levels have following characteristics:

1. Technical system properties, i.e. the technical parameters assessed in the laboratory. Exemplary parameters to assess are technical accuracy, noise, latency, setup time, ideal X-ray exposure, error propagation model.

2. Diagnostic reliability (indirect) and therapeutic reliability (direct), i.e. to access the reliability of a clinical setting in a simulated surgical setup through phantom or cadaver studies. Exemplary parameters for direct assessment are target registration error, safety margins, percentage of resection, cognitive workload, radiation time, system setup time, and time for navigated task.

3. Surgical strategy (indirect) and Surgical performance (direct), i.e. the efficacy in the clinical scenario during first patient trials. The indirect assessment includes the change of strategy and time. Exemplary parameters for direct assessment are cognitive workload, situational awareness, skill acquisition, time, percentage of resection, histological result, pain, usability, X-ray exposure, misplacement detection, preparation time, time for navigated task.

4. Patient outcome, i.e. the effectiveness within a routine clinical scenario evaluated within a multi-site clinical trials or by a meta-analysis. Exemplary parameters for assessment are patient morbidity (recrudescence), pain, cosmetic results, and neurological damage.

1.4 Validation, Verification and Evaluation

5. Economic aspects, i.e. the efficiency of the system that is estimated and assessed during multi-site clinical trials or meta-analysis. Exemplary parameters are cost effectiveness, time reduction, specially trained personal and busy/inactive time of participants.

6. Social, legal, and ethical aspects analyzed using meta models, health care communities and recognized authorities and addresses mainly quality of life issues.

The focus in the interdisciplinary technical and medical research community usually spans from level 1 to level 4. Level 5 is of particular interest for product development, level 6 for market development and the implementation of innovations into the health care system and national treatment guidelines.

Jannin and Korb [106] postulate that the level 1 assessment deals with the intrinsic performance and parameters of a system. This includes all technical parameters of a system. Exemplary studies were performed in the latency and lag of a medical augmented reality system based on a head mounted display [219], the system and subsystem accuracy in the tracking component [27, 42, 99], fiducial registration error [61], and tracking error propagation [13, 215]. Furthermore, the assessment of the system calibration accuracy for a head mounted augmented operating microscope [25] is another examples for assessment of the technical system parameters. Most literature assesses subsystems of image guided surgery systems independently and uses the acquired results to better understand the capacity, limitations, and thus the application domain of the system.

Level 2 deals with the diagnostic and therapeutic reliability [106]. This is often performed with a system setup in a simulated clinical scenario, either in the entire process or a sub process of the surgical task. Exemplary assessments are performed to access the placement accuracy and the required duration to complete a navigated task in phantoms [240, 238] using a head mounted display augmented reality system. Further examples that address the evaluation of their system on the level of the therapeutic reliability was in augmented reality guided needle biopsies [198] and augmented reality based microscope navigation system for neurosurgery [117]. In general on this level the performance parameters in a simulated procedure are assessed. In terms of system accuracy, this is often limited to the assessment of the target registration error as an approximation of the system error [213]. This does however not entirely justify the therapeutic reliability, since this also depends to a large extent on the proper visualization of the information [237]

Level 3 and 4 are assessing the surgical performance, quality and patient outcome either through single center clinical trial, assessing the quality of the treatment and the feasibility (e.g. [50] on level 3) or in a randomized study within multiple centers (e.g. [189] on level 4) to avoid bias in the evaluation.

The entire process of assessing the properties of an image guided surgery system can be derived from health care technology assessment (HTCA) [77]. Standard process there is formalized by a study protocol within ten steps:

1. identify assessment topics,

2. clearly specify assessment problem or question (i.e. assessment objective),

3. determine focus of assessment (e.g. who will perform the assessment),

4. retrieve available evidence,

5. collect new primary data,

6. interpret evidence,

7. synthesize evidence,

8. formulate findings and recommendations,

9. disseminate findings and recommendations,

10. monitor impact.

In general a well designed study protocol and a strict conduction of this protocol including its documentation will ensure on the one side a reliable analysis of the system and on the other side it will save time, money, and resources. Analogue to the software engineering process [40], a proper planning process [38] is the key success for a good and successful assessment.

The study protocol usually includes the assessment objectives, the study conditions, and the details of the method or system. This is again analogue to the software engineering process, i.e. defining the requirements, specifying them and creating the system model. Formal languages like UML can support this process. The conduction of this planned study and its statistical analysis of the assessed data are essential to generate the study report and valid results [106].

In section 5.1 and 5.2 the assessment for to novel systems was performed on level 1 and 2 according to the here described model [106]. Both systems are not yet implemented into clinical trials, but evaluated within simulated procedures. In section 5.3 a new theory is introduced, that uses a model based evaluation of the workflow of the clinically applied procedure and its comparison against the simulated procedure with the new system. For one of the introduced navigation solutions it is studied in details in section 5.3. The results of the study were used to refine the system and prepare a clinical trial. Eventually this could become an inital meta-model for assessment of parameters on level 3 and 4.

CHAPTER 2

Towards Advanced Visualization and Guidance

> Nos quoque oculus eruditos habemus!
> (We, too, have eyes to learn!)
>
> Marcus Tullius Cicero (106-43 BC)

2.1 Towards Complex Image Guided Surgery Systems

The driving forces behind the development and usage of intraoperative navigation and computer assisted systems during therapeutical procedures are on the one hand the increased amount of information that is available during the intervention and on the other hand the motivation to perform an optimal therapy with minimal trauma for the patient. One major challenge within navigated procedures is to present the data intuitively to the physician i.e. spatially and temporally context aware. A successful outcome of a guided intervention in general involves precise planning, e.g. the localization of a specific target region and the execution of this plan e.g. drilling towards a specific target region. This can be relatively easily and intuitively established if there exists a direct line of sight to the target area as in open surgery. With the introduction of less and minimally invasive procedures or the treatment of structures that are not visible in direct vision, the view of the clinician changes from a direct to an indirect view through an endoscope, laparoscope, or other imaging data. Real time imaging data contributes to the accuracy, robustness, and reliability of interventions by enabling views of anatomical and functional informations that are not visible by the human eye. Computer assistance systems make it possible that this information can be seen and related to the clinician's view to support her/his decisions and actions.

The highest accuracy within an intervention is accessible with real time image information. This can be direct vision during open surgery, indirect vision using endoscopic or laparoscopic systems, or any real time medical imaging technology that is capable of simultaneously imaging tools and anatomy. There is no optimal imaging technology for interventions in general and each imaging technology has its specific capabilities and limitations. For anatomical imaging there exist primarily devices based on X-ray and ultrasound technology. Especially the use of ultrasound is a promising technology since it is flexible and non-invasive, but its physical properties and image quality limit its usage. X-ray based imaging such as C-arm and computed tomography imaging is widely used in surgery for diagnosis and therapy, but it is invasive due to ionizing radiation that is applied to the patient and the surgical team.

In trauma and orthopedic surgery the highest accuracy, quality, and safety of procedures can be achieved with the use of intraoperative C-arm or CT fluoroscopy imaging [110]. However, during these procedures the patient and the surgical team are exposed to an additional and considerable amount of ionizing radiation. Within the choice for the optimal treatment, there will be always a balance between high accuracy performance and high amount of radiation exposure during trauma and orthopedic interventions. A perfect placement of implants can be achieved with permanent fluoroscopic imaging. This however also implies a high radiation dose. A major motivation within the development of computer assisted surgery systems in orthopedics and trauma surgery is the reduction of radiation exposure while guaranteeing the optimal patient outcome. Acquiring and presenting the information seamlessly integrated in the clinical workflow will contribute to the decisions and actions of the surgeons in the operating room. Computer assisted surgical procedures will narrow the gap between an average performed surgery and an exceptionally well performed procedure and thus reduce the learning curve of the procedures, especially for novice surgeons.

Traditional application domains for image guided surgery are neurosurgery [193, 78] and trauma or orthopedic surgery [46, 228, 229]. The traditional approach to navigated surgery is to present a single dataset of three-dimensional images and visualize the current position and orientation of a surgical tool in real time within this dataset. It integrates three dimensional imaging data (e.g. computed tomography or magnetic resonance imaging) and spatial localization (tracking) systems and requires tools and methods to estimate their relative transformations. Recent approaches also propose soft tissue navigation. There, the additional challenge of deformable anatomy has to be considered in order to provide a suitable solution. A summary for the motivation of image guided surgery includes

- the abandonment of invasive diagnostic methods, e.g. by reduction of ionizing radiation,

- the pooling of information,

- the improvement of the accuracy, outcome and reliability of a procedure,

- the increase in the safety and robustness of a procedure,

- the full support of real time properties and real time imaging, as well as its integration into the surgcial procedure, and

- the context aware representation of all available anatomical and functional information.

Depending on the requirements for the specific system, these factors have different weights within the final solution for different target applications.

2.2 Towards Full Integration of Patient and Procedure Specific Data

Image guided surgery systems are capable of enhancing the surgeon's visual and mental model by incorporating medical image information and other available patient specific and procedure specific data into her/his surgical procedure using appropriate user interfaces. The availability of this huge amount of information and its fusion for the goal to provide the optimal treatment for the patient has the challenge, not only in engineering of systems, but also in algorithms information processing and information presentation. The amount of information is permanently increasing.

In many of the approaches to design and implement new image guided surgery systems the end user, namely the surgeon, is not included in the development process [230]. Solutions are created using specifications defined by surgeons and engineers, but the development is done solely by engineers. Surgeons using new technologies and imaging systems appear to be adapting their immediate needs to what has been made available to them by engineers and manufacturers. They are devising work-arounds, rather than using advanced technology to improve their surgical work [44]. Navigation solutions often lack a careful analysis and justification of their increased technical complexity compared to state-of-the-art procedures. Its integration and modifications of the current workflow as well as technical, economical and social impacts have to be considered during the design and development of novel image guided surgery solutions. Up to the author's knowledge there is no method available that measures the impact of a newly designed image guided surgery system onto the current clinical workflow. The measure of success for a newly developed system is in general based on a series of phantom, ex-vivo and in-vivo tests after its implementation and setup. Researchers and engineers contribute with their knowledge to the design of smart solutions. Only the process of testing the entire system setup, that can be done after years of algorithm development and engineering work, will justify its clinical value. The number of successful breakthroughs of radical new ideas and technologies are rather low compared to the number of research projects in the field of image guided surgery. In the OR2020 workshop a common sense was that there is a lack of consistent operating room working practices or prescribed workflow routines [44]. The reasons for the missing prescribed workflow routines were identified to be

- the absence of standardized devices and systems,
- the inflexibility of devices and systems,
- the slow and tedious process of switching between applications,
- the inadequate representation of information and data, and
- the unavailability of user-configurable devices and information environment.

The ability to simplify the introduction of new concepts into the everyday surgical routine creates a strong need for an information technology infrastructure and for standards within the operating room [134] in order to design, implement, and analyze new

2.2 Towards Full Integration of Patient and Procedure Specific Data

systems with a surgeon centered approach. This will enable adopted user interfaces and an incorporation of patient and procedure specific data in the right way.

2.3 Towards Minimally Invasive Procedures in Orthopedic Surgery

The major goal of minimally invasive procedures is an efficient target surgery with a minimal iatrogenic trauma, i.e. minimal trauma at the target region and an optimal access route with minimal damage to healthy tissue [149]. The trend towards less invasive procedures is mainly concerning the reduced trauma to soft tissue, which is considered to shorten the recovery time and in general improve the patient outcome. Several studies have shown the superiority of computer assisted techniques in comparison to conventional instrumentation in terms of accuracy and safety in orthopedic surgery [229], especially in percetaneus procedures. Accurately and safely placed implants ensure that there is no occurrence of neurologic deficits and there is no need for repositioning of the implant within a second, additional treatment. However, few studies examine the reduction of invasiveness.

Computer assisted procedures did not always succeed in reducing the invasiveness of the procedures, in particular in orthopedic surgery [129]. Langlotz and Keeve [128] identified three reasons why these surgical procedures have to be invasive in the first place:

- surgeons prefer direct visual access to the region of interest to perform the intervention. This is currently achieved by invasive exposure of the surgical targets through open surgery.

- placements of surgical implants, screws or rods need an access trajectory and proper working volume.

- instruments act upon bony structures and thus need physical contact and open working space for correct positioning as well as easy and safe manipulation.

Whereas reason two and three are subject to improvement of instruments and implants, reason one is subject to a proper navigation system and intraoperative guidance to enable the minimal access route to the target anatomy. However, a proper navigation system and guidance alone cannot enable a less invasive procedure by itself without the enhancement of the instruments and implants. One could solve these issues through design and development of:

a) new instruments for minimally invasive surgery requiring reduced working space,

b) new therapeutic solutions without the direct access requirement, and finally,

c) new and efficient advanced multimodal imaging, display and visualization technology, reducing the need for direct viewing of the anatomy.

Even though the minimally invasiveness of navigated procedures was proposed by the pioneers in computer-assisted surgery it could not be completely established in trauma and orthopedic surgery [129]. Kalfas et al. [111] propose the frameless stereotactic technique that was previously applied in neurosurgical applications to be transferred to the spine

2.3 Towards Minimally Invasive Procedures in Orthopedic Surgery

with similar advantages, i.e. improved accuracy and less invasiveness. Other pioneers like Nolte et al. [177], Merloz et al. [153] and Laine et al. [127] did not reduce the trauma and invasiveness in the first place, but reported improved accuracy and safety in the placement of pedicle screws within the spine surgery procedures.

The two major reasons why the introduced computer assisted approaches could reduce the invasiveness within trauma and orthopedic applications in the past decade were the requirements for precise tracking of the target anatomy and the registration of the target anatomy to preoperative images. For tracking, a reference target is required and it has to be attached to the target anatomy. In general this results in an increased invasiveness in the access route and radiation dose that has to be applied for inserting a reference target into the bone. Furthermore, the registration between the preoperative imaging data and intraoperative navigation system has to be established. In the past this was done by an invasive process of identifying a set of corresponding natural landmarks in the tracking space and image space or matching surfaces.

Recently introduced navigation systems based on intraoperative three dimensional image acquisition and reconstruction in the coordinate frame of the tracking system, so called registration free navigation [52, 79], eliminated the requirement to establish landmarks for registration and, thus, reduced the invasiveness to the attachment of a reference target. The drawback of this technique is however that it introduces an increased amount of ionizing radiation [70, 94] and a three dimensional scan is only possible at distinct points in the operation procedure, e.g. before the intervention for planning or at the end for a confirmation of the proper implant placement. Intraoperative two dimensional fluoroscopic navigation, so called virtual fluoroscopy [63], also eliminates an invasive registration procedure and has only the attachment of a reference frame as an invasive procedure. However, navigation is thereby constrained to a set two dimensional planes and not entirely in three dimensions.

For trauma and orthopedic surgery the method of choice for imaging is in general based on X-ray radiation. In order to ensure less invasive access routes to the target anatomy, in general an increased amount of radiation dose is applied. Since this provides visual feedback and a real time estimate of the relationship between instruments and the target bone region it is an alternative to direct visual access. Current orthopedic and trauma surgery applications are often based on preoperative computed tomography data, intraoperative mobile or stationary C-arms, or CT fluoro imaging in the interventional suites. All of these imaging technologies expose the patient and the surgical team to a huge amount of radiation [35, 70, 94, 190]. The ultimate goal towards minimally invasive surgery, especially for orthopedic and trauma surgery applications, will be navigation solutions that, in addition to less trauma caused by the access route and treatment, optimize the applied radiation dose to a minimum, while ensuring a safe and reliable procedure. This ensures the best and safest patient outcome of the intervention.

CHAPTER 3

Medical Application Domain

> Surgeons must be very careful
> When they take the knife!
> Underneath their fine incisions
> Stirs the Culprit - Life!
>
> *Emily Elizabeth Dickinson (1830-1886)*

3.1 The Spine

Image guided interventions of the spine require anatomical, physiological, and biomechanical knowledge in addition to the indications of fracture and other abnormalities in order to derive the planning and decision steps for the guided intervention. The planning includes the definition of the trajectory of access to the vertebra of interest. Guided procedures in general support access trajectories and treatment at the target area. There are several possibilities for access trajectories depending on the individual anatomical structures, the physiological structure, and the clinical indication.

3.1.1 Spine Anatomy

The human spine consists of 33 bones, 24 vertebrae, 5 sacrum segments and 4 fused coccyx segments. The vertebrae are categorized in 7 cervical (C1-C7), 12 thoracic (T1-T12), and 5 lumbar (L1-L5) elements (cf. figure 3.1) in craniocaudal direction.

The vertebrae of the spine progressively enlarge from the cervical to the lumbar region. There is also a large inter-subject variability in size within the same vertebra level. The size of a vertebra defines the volume. The vertebra with the smallest size and volume is found in the cervical region and the vertebra with the largest in the lumbar. Inter-subject variations are based on gender and general body dimensions.

Medical Application Domain

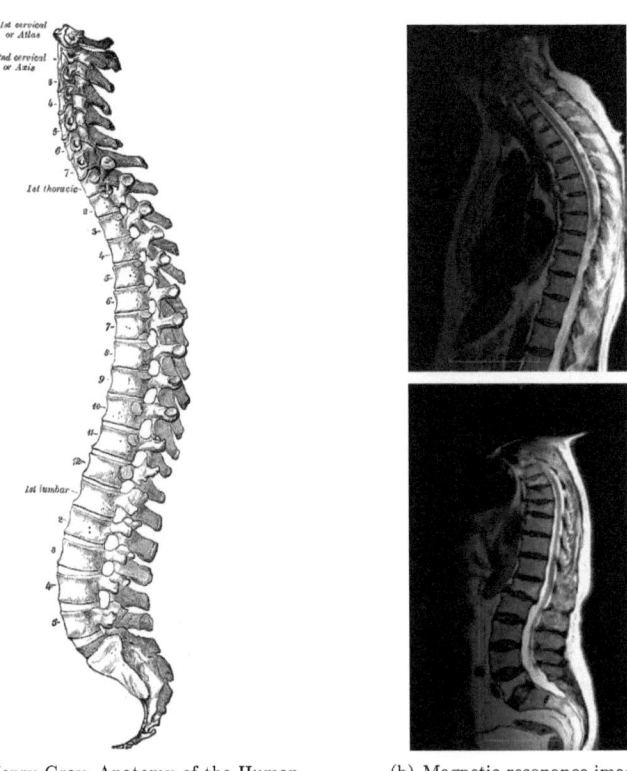

(a) From Henry Gray, Anatomy of the Human Body, 1918, Fig. 111.

(b) Magnetic resonance image.

Figure 3.1: Lateral/Sagittal view of the vertebral column.

3.1 The Spine

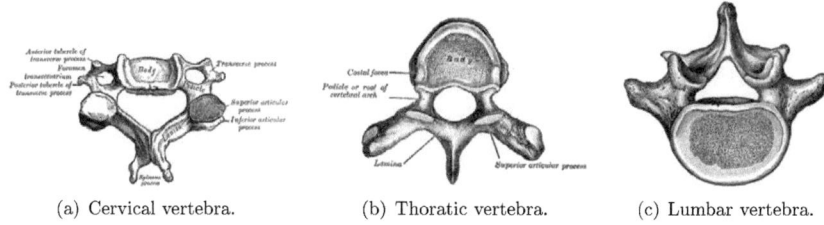

(a) Cervical vertebra.   (b) Thoratic vertebra.   (c) Lumbar vertebra.

Figure 3.2: The difference between cervical, thoratic and lumbar spine. Figures from Henry Gray, Anatomy of the Human Body, 1918, Fig. 82, 84 and 94.

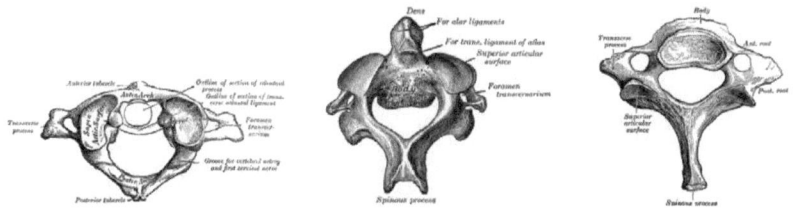

(a) 1st cervical vertebra or atlas.   (b) 2nd cervical vertebra or atlas.   (c) 7th cervical vertebra.

Figure 3.3: The cervical spine shows a huge variation in anatomy from C1 to C7. Figures from Henry Gray, Anatomy of the Human Body, 1918, Fig. 82, 84 and 94.

The cervical spine, located in the neck, has a huge variation from top (C1) to the bottom (C7) (cf. figure 3.3). There is less variation in the thoracic from top (T1) to the bottom (T12) and lumbar spine (L1 - L5). The anatomical deviation in size is especially of importance for the filling volume for vertebroplasty procedures to avoid overfilling. The different orientation of the vertebrae is of special interest to identify the optimal access route.

The spine lies centrally embedded in the human body, covered dorsally by muscles and surrounded ventrally by vital organs and pathways. Its distance from the surface of the skin is smallest in a dorsal direction and largest ventrally and laterally.

3.1.2 Access Trajectories to the Vertebrae

Access principles to the vertebra that are of interest will be granted through various entrances and within different directions. The surgical access route should be least traumatic to minimize the iatrogenic trauma, i.e. the trauma caused by the treatment [149]. A general access route for minimally invasive endoscopic procedures is ventral [17], i.e.

45

access through the anterior direction, or lateral access.

Motivated by the fact that the smallest distance between the surface of the skin and the spine is in dorsal direction, interventions using this access trajectories are desirable to minimize the trauma. Especially transpedicular and parapedicular approaches for fixation of the spine as trauma reduction method or cement augmentation of the spine are widely used procedures.

3.2 Spine Interventions

This section summarizes some of the spine interventions that are proposed to be ideal for the later introduced newly developed navigation systems (sections 4.1 and 4.2). In general percutaneous, dorsal approaches are well suited for the later introduced new solutions. Applications of ventral spinal procedures (cf. section 3.2.1) and their trend towards minimally invasive endoscopic guided procedures are briefly introduced. Interventions for pedicle screw placement for fixation, compression and decompression of the spine (cf. section 3.2.2) and vertebroplasty procedures for cement augmentation of vertebrae along with its instrumentation (cf. section 3.2.3) are described in details since they are primary application domains for the new navigation solutions. Their challenge is to ensure the perfect access route through the pedicle. Other future directions in spine surgery such as disc replacement, bone graft substitutes for fusion, or biologic innovations [200] are not discussed here since they are not in the focus of the proposed navigation systems in chapter 4 in this thesis with major modifications of the current system setup.

3.2.1 Ventral Approach

Minimally invasive endoscopic guided techniques for management of spinal trauma have been established as the standard procedure for many anterior, lateral or medial approached interventions [17]. Chronic pain syndromes in up to 50% of the patient after open access surgery were the motivation for the introduction of less invasive and minimally invasive procedures. The results of a five year study by Beisse et al. [17] show that endoscopic procedures considerably reduce the postoperative pain syndromes. They reported this in a randomized study with 60 patients, 30 patients treated endoscopically and 30 patients treated with open surgery [16]. Amongst the patients treated endoscopically they reported a reduction in the duration of administration of analgesics (31%) and the overall dose (42%) in comparison with the patients who received open surgery treatment. 80% of the patients treated by the minimally invasive endoscopic procedure returned to their previous employment. Furthermore, endoscopic procedures can be compared in operation duration and complication rate with open access surgery. Another advantage of endoscopic surgery is the lower risk of infection due to less inflicted tissue and reduced tissue exposure time for infection during surgery. This study shows the high motivation to further facilitate minimally invasive procedures in spine surgery.

3.2.2 Dorsal Approach - Pedicle Screw Placements

Transpedicular fixation became a standard procedure for vertebral fractures, even so for various interventions combined techniques with ventral approaches are recommended [119]. The so called posterior or dorsal instrumentation uses the dorsal access route to the spine and ideally places the screw such, that it uses the whole diameter of the isthmus of the pedicle. In general this procedure is performed under permanent fluoroscopic control usually in two planes, the anterior-posterior and lateral. To mark the entry into the pedicle and to open it often a needle or awl is inserted under fluoroscopy control. On the anterior-posterior X-ray view the needle tip should not touch the medial curve of the pedicle, which forms the wall of spinal canal and its pathway. On the lateral view the needle should be parallel to the superior and inferior edge of the pedicle. Alternative to the needle or awl, automatic drilling devices be used in order to open the pedicle for screw insertion. After confirmation of the perfect placement of the supporting tool (needle/Kirschner-Wire) the screw is placed. Using special equipment the pedicle screw is placed, either guided by the placed Kirschner-Wire and by lateral X-ray imaging or only lateral imaging to control that no perforation of the vertebra in anterior direction towards the aorta occurs. Once the screw is placed, plates are inserted for fixation, compression or decompression of the spine. The process after the placement of the guiding tool is performed often by the support of clever mechanical construction of devices, wires, and screws. X-ray imaging is in general only applied to confirm the correct placement. The challenge for navigation is within the initial placement of a guiding wire or supporting tool into its optimal position and orientation through the pedicle.

3.2.3 Dorsal Approach - Vertebroplasty

Vertebroplasty provides a minimal-invasive surgical technique for the cement augmentation of vertebral bodies following osteoporotic compression fractures or malignant processes [148, 191]. The procedure is performed percutaneously, i.e. through a small incision point in the skin. In comparison to non-percutaneous techniques, where the skin and tissue is removed to enable access to the bone, percutaneous procedures insert only a needle or guiding wire through the skin. The process involves the dorsal insertion of a Kirschner-Wire (cf. figure 3.4(a)) or a needle (e.g. Jamshidi needle), in general supported using fluoro CT (cf. figure 3.4(b)) or X-ray images by C-arms. In case of a Kirschner-Wire, once an accurate placement is confirmed (e.g. through a spiral computed tomography scan), a canula is inserted and positioned (cf. figure 3.4(c)). The canula is inserted also under imaging control i.e. fluoro CT (cf. figure 3.5) or X-ray image control. The instrumentation for cement augmentation is inserted through the needle or canula. The cement is filled into the bone again under CT fluoro (cf. figure 3.6) or X-ray image control. The final augmentation result is confirmed during the intervention with a spiral CT scan (cf. figure 3.7(b)), multiplanar X-ray images, or a 3D reconstruction by a C-arm. Kyphoplasty has been developed as an advancement of vertebroplasty that enables the decompression of the fractured bone using a balloon. The cement filling is applied within the balloon. Thus its shape is a sphere and it is questionable if the biomechanical consistency is sufficient. New methods are released using the approach of kyphoplasty with the possibility of filling

Medical Application Domain

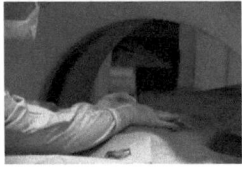 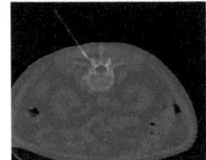 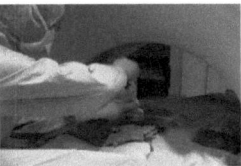

(a) Kirschner wire insertion.　(b) Kirschner wire in fluoro CT image.　(c) Canula insertion.

Figure 3.4: Insertion of a Kirschner wire and canula for cement augmentation during a vertebroplasty intervention. Pictures talken during an intervention at Klinikum Innenstadt, Munich by Prof. K.J. Pfeifer and Prof. E. Euler, 2005.

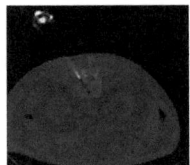 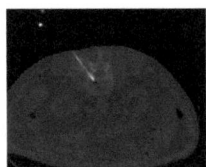 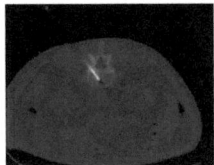

(a) Beginning of canula insertion.　(b) Intermediate control image.　(c) Final placement.

Figure 3.5: CT images of canula insertion for cement augmentation during a vertebroplasty intervention. Pictures from an intervention at Klinikum Innenstadt, Munich by Prof. K.J. Pfeifer and Prof. E. Euler, 2005.

the cement such, that it has a more natural distribution within the cavity of the vertebra.

3.3 Computer Assisted Spine Interventions

In the past two decades computer assisted surgery systems were introduced into the operation room [184], after their advent in neurosurgery in the early 80s [114, 74], applications for spine surgery in the early 90s [147, 150] and later various other orthopedics and trauma surgery [228, 229] were introduced. Driving motivations for the introduction of computer assisted surgery systems are

- reduction of invasiveness e.g. by optimizing the access route, minimizing ionizing radiation and reducing the unnecessary damages to neighboring tissues,

- increase of safety and reliability of therapy e.g. by improving intervention accuracy, visualizing critical organs and detections of human errors as early as possible in the surgical process,

3.3 Computer Assisted Spine Interventions

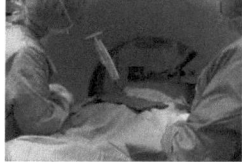
(a) Instrumentation for cement augmentation.

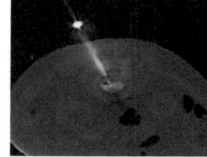
(b) Fluoro CT during filling.

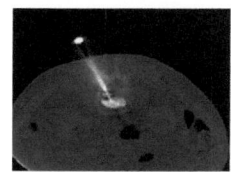
(c) Fluoro CT for filling confirmation.

Figure 3.6: Process of cement augmentation during a vertebroplasty intervention. Pictures from an intervention at Klinikum Innenstadt, Munich by Prof. K.J. Pfeifer and Prof. E. Euler, 2005.

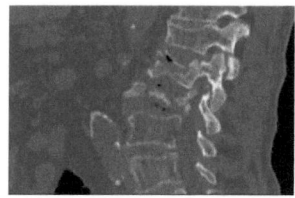
(a) Pre-interventional CT scan for diagnosis and planning.

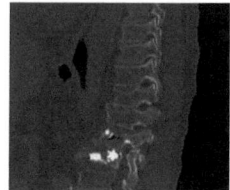
(b) Post interventional control scan.

Figure 3.7: Sagittal intersection pre- and post-interventional spiral CT scans of the inflicted vertebral column T12/L1. Pictures from an intervention at Klinikum Innenstadt, Munich by Prof. K.J. Pfeifer and Prof. E. Euler, 2005.

- introduction of novel interventions e.g. by definition of new non invasive interventions which are only possible under precise navigation and multi-modal imaging.

The ultimate goal of all systems is to improve the patient outcome by an optimal intervention. This includes narrowing the gap between an exceptional well performed intervention and an average intervention. Image guided interventions are supposed to guaranty an exceptional outcome of the intervention. However computer assisted procedures did not always succeed in reducing the invasiveness of the procedures, in particular in orthopedic surgery [129]. Langlotz and Keeve [128] identified three reasons why these surgical procedures have to be invasive in the first place:

- surgeons prefer direct visual access to the region of interest to perform the intervention. This is currently achieved by invasive exposure of the surgical targets through open surgery.
- placements of surgical implants, screws or rods need an access trajectory and proper working volume.
- instruments act upon bony structures and thus need physical contact and open working space for correct positioning as well as easy and safe manipulation.

Whereas the latter reasons are subject of improving instruments and implants, the first reason is subject to a proper navigation system and intraoperative guidance to enable the minimal access route to the target anatomy and it involves the development of appropriate imaging, tracking, displays, and visualization techniques. One could attack all above mentioned issues through design and development of:

a) new instruments for minimally invasive surgery requiring reduced working space,

b) new therapeutic solutions without the direct access requirement, and finally,

c) new and efficient advanced multimodal imaging, display and visualization technology, reducing the need for direct viewing of the anatomy.

In this thesis the focus is on the latter, aiming at providing new navigation and visualization solutions for computer assisted minimally invasive surgery.

3.3.1 History of Computer Assisted Spinal Interventions

The first reported approach in computer assisted spine surgery was adopted from stereotactic neurosurgery. Brodwater et al. [37] used an operation microscope for a spine intervention, but instead of the rigid stereotactic frame they attached external markers to the skin of the patient. The measured error was extremely large, 28.81 mm (SD 7.49) in the disc space localization. They could not find a relating motion pattern between skin markers and the spine anatomy, thus they were not able to decrease the error. Roessler et al. [194] confirmed that the use of skin markers exceed the accuracy required for navigated surgery in the spine. Within their studies they report an application accuracy of 11.3 mm mean (range 5-20mm) on real patients. Based on the outcome of this studies, further

3.3 Computer Assisted Spine Interventions

development in computer assisted spinal interventions proposed the use of dynamic reference target (DRB) [177], a rigid target that is attached to the bone of interest, i.e. the vertebra to be treated. This provides a good, however, an invasive reference system. The registration relative to that reference frame is performed by corresponding points or features between image and tracking space [129]. The attachment of the dynamic reference base avoids errors caused by patient motion and deformation of the spine. It has been proven to be superior in terms of accuracy over skin markers.

Navigated interventions were extended to various other orthopedic and trauma surgery disciplines including hip arthroplasty and knee arthroplasty [4]. Computer assisted surgery contributes also to the enhancement within these application domains.

The currently available computer assisted system for the spine can be categorized by the used imaging technology in:

- CT based navigation (cf. section 3.3.1.1),

- two dimensional C-arm/Fluoro guided (cf. section 3.3.2), and

- three dimensional reconstructed C-arm based navigation (cf. section 3.3.3).

The different approaches were compared in multiple studies. A summary is provided in section 3.3.3.1 later in this chapter. There are commercially available solutions for navigated spine surgery. VectorVision® spine by BrainLAB AG (http://www.brainlab.com), that enables navigation based on preoperative CT and intraoperative fluoroscopic images simultaneously. Similar to this system, the Synergy™Experience StealthStation® System by Medtronics (http://www.medtronicnavigation.com/) provides a full suite including two-dimensional and three-dimensional C-arm as well as CT based navigation. Another available, complete system for navigated spine surgery is Navitrack® FluoroSpine® by ORTHOsoft (http://www.orthosoft.ca).

3.3.1.1 Preoperative CT Navigation with External Tracking

General principles of CT based navigation is summarized by Jaramaz et al. [110]. This approach to navigated spine surgery is based on the usage of preoperative acquired CT data, the placement of a dynamic reference base into the therapeutic target anatomy (i.e. vertebra of interest), the registration of the CT data within the spatial localization coordinate system (e.g. optical tracking), and the visualization of the tracked instruments within the CT data as multiplanar reconstructions. Visionary systems propose augmented reality techniques for the in-situ visualization of the navigation information based on preoperative CT scans [22, 30]. Special motivation for CT based navigation is in the cervical spine [252] where additional critical structures like vertebral artery, spinal nerve, or spinal cord are nearby and thus at higher risk compared to the lumbar spine region. Laine et al. [126] conduced a randomized study with 100 patients for comparison of the accuracy within screw insertion with and without computer assistance based on preoperative CT data. For both, the navigated and the conventional method, a preoperative spiral CT scan was acquired and in case of the computer assisted insertion the three dimensional scan

Medical Application Domain

was registered intraoperatively with the navigation system SurgiGATE Spine (Medivision, Oberdorf, Switzerland) that was already evaluated earlier by the same group within a prospective clinical trial within 30 patients [127]. Their conclusion of the randomized studies was that computer assisted procedures are more accurate and reliable. They derive this conclusion from the percentage of pedicle perforation by the placed screws with both methods. They reported 13.4% (37 of 277 screws) perforation within the conventional procedure and only 4.6% (10 of 219 screws) in the computer assisted procedure. Amiot et al. [3] performed a comparative study of 150 patients, 100 treated with conventional method and 50 treated with computer assistance based on preinterventional CT data and intraoperative navigation. With computer assistance 5.4% of the screws were placed in a not ideal position. In contrast, the control group that was treated with the conventional method had 15.3% of screws placed in a not ideal position. Furthermore, none of the patients treated with computer assistance had to undergo reoperation and no long term neurologic deficits occurred in contrast to the control group that was treated conventionally, where seven patients had to undergo reoperation and four reported long term neurologic deficits. Geerling at al. [71] summarized various studies showing that the misplacement rate using CT based navigation systems is extremely low [3, 75, 112, 126, 209], especially compared to not navigated, conventional procedures.

The unique part within preoperative CT based navigation in spine surgery is the registration of CT data with the tracking coordinate system. The first attempts adopted from stereotactic neurosurgery showed that point based registration of fiducials attached to the skin are not sufficient in terms of the target registration error [37, 194]. The introduction of reference frames rigidly attached to the vertebra of interest and registration methods based on surface registration reduced the target registration error significantly [129]. In general an initial point based registration method is iteratively refined by surface registration between the extracted vertebra surface in the CT scan and digitalized surface points in the tracking space. One exemplary method is the iterative closest point algorithm (ICP) [20, 265]. For an acceptable result using surface registration methods the acquired points should be widely distributed over the intraoperative accessible anatomy [176]. However, the method for the acquisition of surface points for registration in the tracking coordinate frame requires an invasive procedure. This is one of the major reasons, why Langlotz and Keeve [128] state that the navigated procedures did not reduce the invasiveness in the first place, but the robustness and reliability of its outcome in terms of placement accuracy. An novel approach for registration of CT data is based on a unscented Kalman Filter (UKF) between CT data and tracked ultrasound [158]. According to Gebhard et al. [69] another limitation besides the invasive registration process is that the CT reflects the preoperative anatomical status and is only applicable with intact vertebral bodies and assuming the anatomical situation did not change between the data acquisition and its intraoperative usage e.g. by compression or decompression. Slomczykowski et al. [221] show that the radiation dose of a preoperative required CT for navigated surgery exceeds the radiation dose applied during fluoroscopic navigation.

Commercially available systems based on preoperative CT data advertise the possibility of optimal screw placement throughout the entire spine, reduction of radiation exposure, increasing efficiencies, and a minimal invasive approach for reduced recovery times.

3.3.2 2D C-arm/Fluoroscopy Guidance

The navigation based on fluoroscopic C-arm images and external tracking, often referred to as virtual fluoroscopy was introduced in parallel by Nolte et al. [175] and Foley et al. [62, 63]. The procedure does not require preoperative imaging data and an invasive registration procedure. Further advantages are the availability of a fluoroscopic imaging device that is capable of imaging the recent anatomical situation and can provide updates any time.

Within the procedure a reference frame, identical to CT based navigation is attached to the vertebra of interest under fluoroscopic control. The navigation with the fluoroscopic C-arm images is not based on a three dimensional dataset, but on 2D fluoroscopic images. The C-arm is tracked in the same coordinate system than the dynamic reference base within the vertebra and the instruments. Modeling the C-arm geometry using a camera model and projections (cf. figure 4.11), the position of the instruments can be projected in any image of an arbitrary positioned C-arm. In general an anterior-posterior and a lateral image are used for 2D fluoroscopic navigation [64].

One challenge in fluoroscopic based navigation is its two dimensional nature and thus a navigation in not in all three dimensions, but only two dimensional projective images. Another challenge is the X-ray geometric distortion and its online correction [140]. In general a ring containing X-ray markers on two different planes is attached to the image detector for online distortion correction [47]. Furthermore, the ring consists of tracking markers to be localized by the optical tracking system. The misplacement rate of implants using 2D fluoroscopic navigation was classified to be similar to the misplacement rate in CT based navigation in the spine [64].

3.3.3 Three Dimensional Recoconstructed C-arm Guidance

The underlying concept of this technique is the intraoperative 3D cone-beam reconstruction using a mobile C-arm [192]. The C-arm is extended by markers for an optical tracking system. During the acquisition the C-arm rotates around its iso-center with over 180 degrees. The reconstructed volume is, after a one time calibration routine, known within the coordinate system of the optical tracking system. This enables a direct reference and thus visualization of the tracked instruments within the reconstructed volume without any registration procedure. The limitation is however that this is not a real time imaging technology in contrast to the 2D fluoroscopic imaging. A three dimensional scan is only performed at very distinct points during the intervention, i.e. at the beginning to acquire imaging data for three dimensional navigation or at the end to confirm the correct placement during the surgery. In twelve patients Euler et al. [52] showed a sufficient accuracy of this procedure for the placement of pedicle screws. Its usage is superior to navigation based on preoperative computed tomography data, mainly because of a non invasive registration method (i.e. registration free) and more up to date three dimensional imaging data.

Medical Application Domain

3.3.3.1 Discussion of Different Approaches for Navigated Spine Surgery

Holly [96, 97] compares the three different approaches for computer assisted spine surgery based on CT data, intraoperative cone-beam reconstruction, and 2D fluoroscopy. In general both 3D navigation methods have the advantage of navigating the instruments in all three dimensions and thus give correct guidance information. Their major drawback is that both procedures do not provide real time imaging during the intervention. A rescan in case the anatomy moves or deforms is not easily possible. Especially in case of CT based navigation the image data set reflects a preoperative situation and assumes that the target anatomy does not change until the treatment. Furthermore, CT based navigation has the major disadvantage of an invasive procedure for registration, i.e. digitalizing points in the tracking coordinate system. Navigated 2D fluoroscopy showed promising results, however, it is limited to a number of 2D projections.

There exist several interventional spinal procedures that treat the vertebra through one single or both pedicles from dorsal, which can be supported by the above introduced navigation procedure. The procedures are mainly fracture trauma reduction in form of cement augmentation of the vertebra (vertebroplasty and kyphoplasty), compression, decompression, and fusion or fixation with pedicle screws. All pedicle approaches require precise guidance to place the channel through the pedicle without any perforation, especially in medial direction, i.e. the direction towards the spinal court. Comparing the accuracy of conventional non navigated to any navigated procedures in the spine the placement accuracy can be significantly improved [3, 75, 112, 122, 126, 189, 209]. In general the pedicles are classified in their ideal position and deviation of this position in medial and lateral direction. A method to clinically classify the placement of pedicle screw depending on the level on its perforation was described by Arand et al. [6, 7]. They distinguish between level A, a central position of the screw without any perforation, level B that describes the group that has lateral/medial or cranial/caudal perforation smaller than the thread of the screw, and level C with pedicle perforation higher than the thread of the screw.

All the above listed papers show that computer assisted procedures in general improved the outcome of surgery in terms of placement accuracy. However, no obvious clinical advantage could be established in the past [208]. Schulze et al. showed that neurologic symptoms are rarely influenced by an eccentric pedicle screw tract. There was no variation in the syndromes even for penetration of the pedicle wall with up to 6 mm [208]. Navigation in the spine, however, will never replace the profound anatomical and physiological knowledge of the surgeon about the target anatomy [64].

CHAPTER 4

Two Novel Approaches to Image Guided Surgery

> *If you don't know where you are going, any road will do.*
> *Chinese proverb*
>
> *If you don't know where you are, a map won't help.*
> *Watts S. Humphrey*

4.1 Hybrid Augmented Reality Navigation Interface

My first approach for improving the navigation during percutaneous spinal interventions is the use of a head mounted display based augmented reality system [238, 240]. The usage of in-situ visualization is motivated by many applications where the surgeon has to relate the medical imaging data to the operation situs (cf. figure 4.1).

Within this section I will explain the system setup including its components and calibration in detail and discuss its limitations. Furthermore, the newly developed advanced visualization concepts towards the application for pedicle screw placement are described. A head mounted display based augmented reality system that is extended by new visualization concepts adopted from traditional multiplanar reconstructed slice navigation. Experiments and results of the technical system parameters, as well as the results of simulated surgical procedures are presented in section 5.1.

4.1.1 Related Work in Head Mounted Display Based Augmented Reality

Augmented reality was proposed for surgery as an alternative visualization method to traditional multiplanar reconstructed slice navigation. In orthopedics it is applicable for training, planning, and interventions [30]. The significant differences of an augmented re-

Two Novel Approaches to Image Guided Surgery

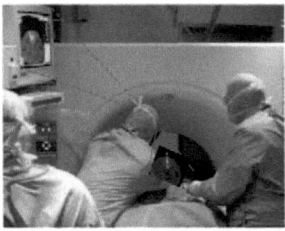
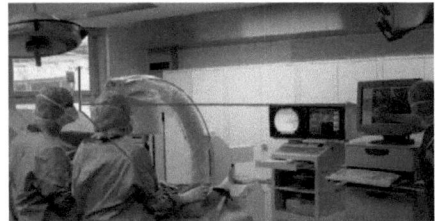

(a) CT navigated intervention.   (b) C-arm navigated operation.

Figure 4.1: The surgeons are relating the information presented on a monitor to the operation situs. In the left image the CT slice was added to the image to show an exemplary solution for a better visualization.

ality system compared to standard, monitor based navigation are the display techniques and visualization, which results in a more intuitive human interface interaction. For medical imaging, tracking, and registration exactly the same or similar devices and methods are used, compared to general image guided surgery applications. As open issues in augmented reality research Blackwell et al. [30] identify the line of sight requirement of the tracking, non rigid registration, and intraoperative updates of images. These issues are however not specific to augmented reality visualization, but image guided surgery in general. Alternative solutions were developed over the past ten years to overcome some of these limitations. Specific research issues dedicated to medical augmented reality are the display technology, user interface, depth perception, and synchronization of image and tracking data. One of the first medical augmented reality systems, that is based on a head mounted display system, was proposed by Bajura et al. [12]. They augmented the image of a video camera with a spatially registered ultrasound image and visualized it in a video see-through head mounted display. Another application using a video see-through head mounted display was proposed by Fuchs et al. [66] to display the images of a laparoscope through synthetic windows directly onto the patient. Sauer et al. [206] developed a video see through head mounted display system for multipurpose usage. Exemplary applications are the visualization of fMRI for neurosurgery [202], ultrasound guidance [203], CT based navigation [204], and MRI based needle biopsies [248]. A clone of their system was used in this work. The system setup is explained in the following sections.

4.1.2 System Components

The system is a combination of two existing components, the three dimensional user interface RAMP [206] and an optical tracking system. A system was developed for procedures that is based on a computed tomography scan. Before the computed tomography scan fiducials were attached. These markers are visible simultaneously in computed tomography and tracking space (cf. figure 4.2). This allows using the proposed visualization on any object, provided that fiducials are attached to it before the computed tomography scan. Any other patient to modality registration will be also suitable for the introduced

4.1 Hybrid Augmented Reality Navigation Interface

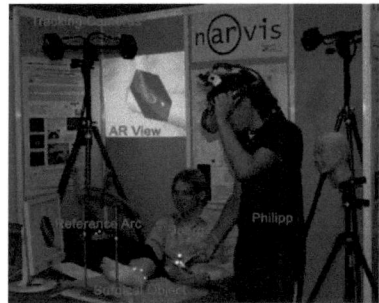
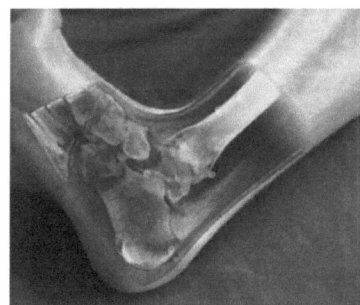

(a) System overview.   (b) Augmented, volume rendered CT data.

Figure 4.2: The head mounted display augmented reality system presented at DGU in Berlin 2005.

system, as long as the combined fiducials are visible by the respective modality.

4.1.2.1 Hardware Setup

The augmented reality system is based on a stereoscopic video see-through head mounted display and was developed by Sauer et al. (SCR, Princeton, USA) [202]. The head mounted display, a ProView from Kaiser Electro-Optics Inc. (Ann Arbor, MI, USA) with an resolution of 1024×768, is equipped with two color cameras with a resolution of 640×480 to obtain images of the real world and display these images on the miniature displays. Additionally, a tracking camera is attached to the system for head pose estimation [206]. This technique, often referred to as inside-out tracking, has been proven to minimize the error of visualization in the viewing direction in augmented reality [92]. The tracking camera consists of a black and white camera with an attached infrared filter and a ring of LEDs around the lens of the camera.

There are two reasons for the usage of a video see-through display (i.e. the real world is imaged by video cameras and visualized on a head mounted display) over an optical see-through device (i.e. the real world is seen directly through a half transparent plate that is capable to display also the virtual data). Firstly, video see-through systems achieve a perfect temporal synchronization of video data and head pose data since the cameras within that setup are genlocked, eliminating any time lag between the images of visualization and tracking camera. Non optimal temporal synchronization can lead to perceivable jitter or swimming [204]. Secondly, in video see-through head mounted displays the developer has more options for visualization since he/she has full control over the real world image. This includes the possibility to apply image processing methods to the video images.. In optical systems only manipulation of the virtual image, e.g. brightening of the augmentation, is possible.

The drawback of using a single camera system for instrument tracking is that large marker configurations are needed for a precise localization of targets [247]. As large tracking targets attached to instruments are not desired in the operating theatre, an external optical tracking system is applied. The ARTtrack1 (Advanced Realtime Tracking GmbH, Weilheim, Germany) is used in the setup to track instruments and the surgical region of interest. A marker frame (cf. figure 4.3(D)) is used to establish a common coordinate frame between the inside-out and external optical tracking system. The hardware setup is shown in figure 4.3.

The transformation from the coordinate system of the external tracking device to the two dimensional coordinates in the image coordinates is given by

$$^{Overlay}H_{Target} = {}^{Overlay}H_{Cam} \; {}^{Cam}H_{Frame} \left({}^{Ext}H_{Frame}\right)^{-1} {}^{Ext}H_{Target}, \qquad (4.1)$$

where the transformations $^{Ext}H_{Frame}$ and $^{Ext}H_{Target}$ are provided by the external tracking system for the pose of the tracking frame and the surgical region of interest. $^{Cam}H_{Frame}$ and $^{Overlay}H_{Cam}$ are derived using Tsai camera calibration [242] and model the extrinsic and intrinsic camera parameters. Figure 4.4 shows an overview of all involved transformations and coordinate systems.

4.1.3 Phantom Design and Clinical Integration

The core requirement for a navigation solution in trauma surgery is its seamless integration into the clinical workflow and, to a large extent, an automatic configuration with no additional interactive calibration or registration procedures during surgery.

Most methods described in literature use tracked pointers to register markers in patient space with their corresponding centroids segmented from imaging data e.g. [117]. As shown in section 3.3.1, dynamic reference base, i.e. a target rigidly attached to the anatomy of interest, provides the most accurate procedure and incorporates an invasive procedure for registration. If the target is attached before the scan, which is only possible in combination with intra-operative imaging technologies, the procedure will be registration free. A promising trend in image guided interventions are systems that enable intraoperative imaging co-registered by construction or by a one time calibration with the tracking coordinate system.

For our phantom experiments we designed markers that are automatically detectable in the CT imaging data and in the physical space by the optical tracking system. We use CT-Spots (4 [mm] diameter) from Beekley Corp (Bristol, CT, USA) coated with infrared retro reflective material (cf. figure 4.3(E)). This provides a completely automatic registration procedure for our phantom. This technique will be however questionable within real patients for spine surgery, since skin markers were proven not to provide sufficient accuracy [37, 194]. An ideal solution for the registration is either the usage of intraoperative imaging data or the attachment of a reference target into the vertebra of interest before computed tomography or alternative preoperative imaging. For our phantom however, we used these combined markers attached to the surface of the phantom, which is a rigid structure and does not move or deform with respect to the target area.

Following the approach of Wang et al. [249], an automatic segmentation is used, based on binary thresholding and region growing, followed by a classification of the segmented

4.1 Hybrid Augmented Reality Navigation Interface

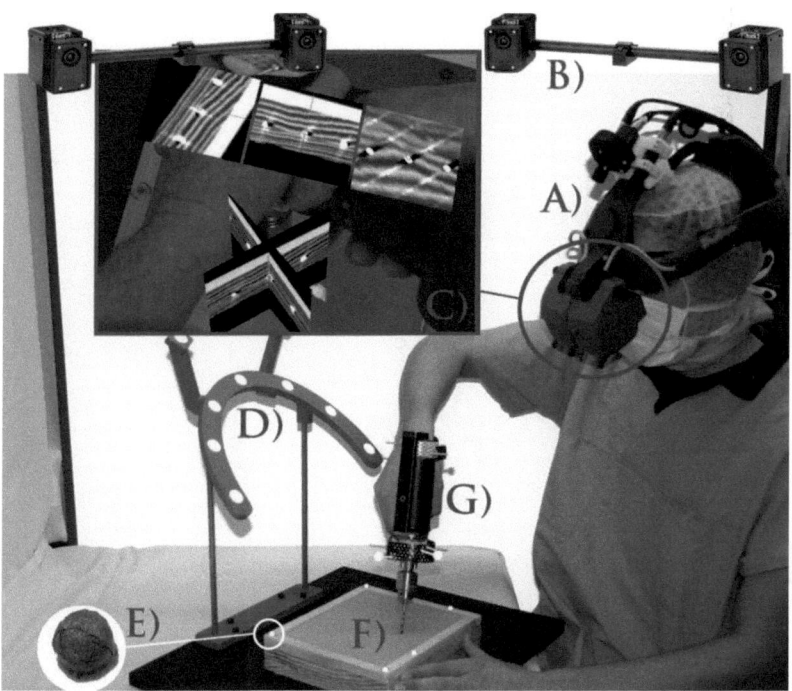

Figure 4.3: Illustration of the setup for the hybrid navigation interface. (A) The HMD with two cameras for the video images and a single camera tracker for determination of the pose relative to the marker frame (D). An external optical infrared tracking device (B) is used for tracking surgical instruments (G) and CT detectable, infrared retro-reflective markers (E) attached to the phantom (F). The hybrid navigation view (C) is displayed on two miniature LCD monitors. In this augmentation all coordinate systems are visualized representing the transformations involved. The marker frame (D) is used as a common coordinate system for both, single camera tracking (A) and external optical tracking (B).

Two Novel Approaches to Image Guided Surgery

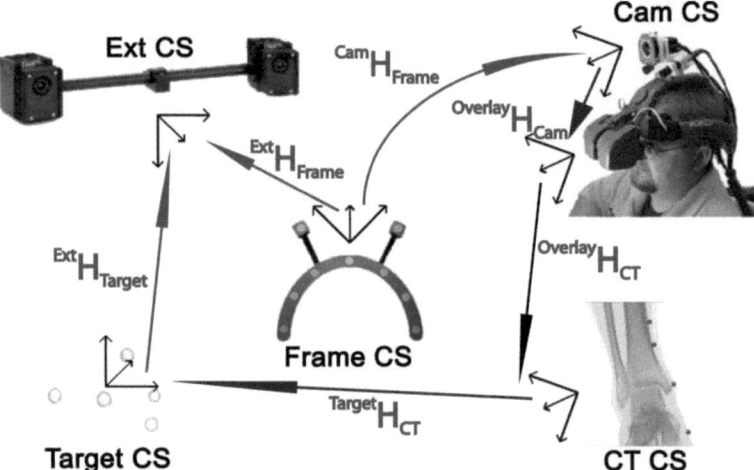

Figure 4.4: The coordinate systems and transformations within the head mounted display augmented reality system. The red arrows indicate tracking data that are updated multiple times in a second. The blue arrows indicate transformations that are estimated by a one time calibration or registration. The black arrow indicates a transformation that is a concatenation of several transformations (cf. equation 4.2)

region. The centroids of segmented regions are calculated intensity-weighted using the voxel intensities of the imaging data.

Finally, the correct point correspondences are established and the transformation $^{Target}H_{CT}$ from the CT coordinates into the tracking coordinates is computed. The correspondence is established by a distance-weighted graph matching approach [76] followed by a standard point based registration algorithm [244] minimizing the error $\epsilon = \sum_{i=1}^{n} \left\| p_{Target,i} - {}^{Target}H_{CT} p_{CT,i} \right\|$, where $p_{CT,i}$ are the centroids in the computed tomography coordinate system and $p_{Target,i}$ the three dimensional centroids in the tracking coordinate system. Thus the data in the CT coordinate system can be transformed to the overlay image coordinate system by

$$^{Overlay}H_{CT} = {}^{Overlay}H_{Target} \; {}^{Target}H_{CT}, \qquad (4.2)$$

with $^{Overlay}H_{Target}$ computed as shown in equation 4.1.

4.1.4 Visualization Modes

4.1.4.1 Standard Slice Based Navigation

In standard slice based navigation systems, image data are presented on two dimensional monitors [152, 153]. The displayed slices are controlled by the pose of the instrument. In general this is decomposed into the visualization of the instrument tip and the instrument axis. The position of the instrument tip is computed within the computed tomography coordinates. The three orthogonal slices (axial, frontal, and sagittal) that intersect at the tip of the instrument are computed and rendered in real time. A crosshair indicates the tip of the instrument in each rendered image.

Instead of axial, frontal, and sagittal slices, for rigid and straight instruments two orthogonal slices that intersect in the axis of the instrument are rendered (pseudo sagittal and pseudo axial) to visualize the axis of the instrument. A third plane that is orthogonal to the axis of the instrument and intersects the instrument in its tip is rendered. This standard slice based navigation was implemented in our in-situ visualization software to have all navigation modes available in one single user interface, the head mounted display. Therefore, we project the three orthogonal rendered slices at a fixed location in space in close vicinity to the region of interest (cf. figure 4.5(d)).

4.1.4.2 Augmented Reality Visualization Modes

We implemented various augmented reality visualization modes. The requirement for navigation is the guidance of surgical instruments to a specific target point based on three dimensional imaging data. The requirement for the clinical integration is that no interaction is required to prepare the data (e.g. interactive segmentation or planning). All three implemented augmented reality navigation modes work directly on the DICOM data with the imaging data registered.

Two Novel Approaches to Image Guided Surgery

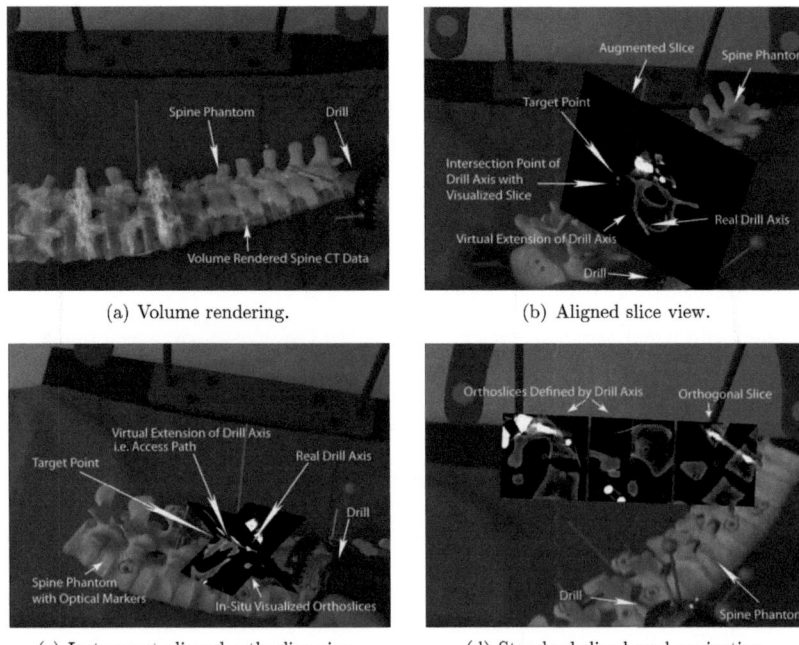

(a) Volume rendering.

(b) Aligned slice view.

(c) Instrument aligned orthoslice view.

(d) Standard slice based navigation.

Figure 4.5: Different visualization modes for navigation that are displayed on the head mounted display.

4.1 Hybrid Augmented Reality Navigation Interface

Volume Rendering: A direct volume rendering technique was implemented, which is a commonly used 2D projective representation method for three dimensional medical imaging data. Intensity values in the volume domain are mapped to the three-dimensional color space and opacity using transfer functions in order to accentuate anatomically interesting structures [80]. In addition to rendering the CT data, a virtual extension of the instrument into the target anatomy is also visualized (cf. figure 4.5(a)).

Slice Based Visualization Modes for In-situ Visualization: In order to improve the performance of surgeons using in-situ visualization for image guided surgery, the concept of standard slice based navigation was adopted. Slice representation is the most commonly used visualization of 3D data for diagnosis, especially by radiologists, but also more and more by surgeons to plan and guide their surgical procedures. It reduces the dimensionality of the three dimensional dataset to a two dimensional representation showing only one or a limited number of planar reconstructions of the data volume. Traditionally, sagittal, coronal (also referred to as frontal), and axial planes are presented. These planes are defined by the patient anatomy and encoded within the DICOM standard. However, any arbitrary plane through the CT volume can be visualized as a two dimensional slice. As an enhancement for in-situ visualization, we use representation methods that are based on visualization of slices through the volume that are spatially aligned with the real patient within the head mounted display. The slices are either defined by the coordinate system of the image data or by the drill axis, as described in the next two paragraphs.

Target Point Aligned Slice View: The first method that is based on slice rendering defines the slice by a point, i.e. the target point of the anatomy and a normal, i.e. one of the base axis of the CT data set, where the direction is closest to the direction of the instrument. Since in our AR rendering system we do not separate real from virtual data and do not support occlusion detection of real objects by their virtual superimposition, the real drill axis is in general entirely occluded by this slice. Thus, a virtual representation of the drill is augmented onto the slice along with the virtual extension of the axis of the drill that shows the access path. The intersection of the virtual extension with the visualized slice defined by the target region is highlighted and is the major feedback for guiding the drill into the defined target region. Practically, the surgeon has to align this point of intersection with the defined target point. The advantage is that the surgeon sees a stable, standard and commonly used slice view. The main drawback of this in-situ visualization method is that the direct vision including the view of the real drill is occluded by the rendered slice (cf. figure 4.5(b)). Recently new rendering techniques were proposed to over come this limitation by context specific and hot spot visualization that enables only an superimposition within a small region of interest.

Instrument Aligned Ortho-Slice In-situ Visualization: An orthoslice view is rendered spatially aligned along the instrument axis. The slices are controlled by the pose of the instrument. The intersection of the two planes corresponds to the instrument axis. Along this line the user can see the extension of the instrument inside the anatomy.

63

4.1.4.3 Hybrid Navigation Interface

To combine the advantages of both systems, a novel hybrid navigation solution is proposed. The hybrid navigation interface fuses the standard, multiplanar reconstruction (MPR) and the above described in-situ visualization methods into a single three dimensional interface (cf. figure 4.6). The MPR is rendered on a virtual plane directly beside the real surgical object. Visualizing this close to the surgical object makes it visible at the same time as the in-situ visualization. The advantage of the in-situ visualization, i.e. intuitive and accurate guidance for lateral dimensions is complemented by the advantages of the MPR method i.e. high accuracy in all three dimensions. Especially the instrument aligned ortho-slice in-situ visualization in combination with the MPR realized within the same HMD proves to be a promising method for the navigation tasks. Experiments show that it is almost as accurate as only MPR and that it is performed in about the same time as the in-situ visualization (cf. table 5.1). The major advantage reported by the surgeons that conducted the experiments was that exactly the same slices are rendered twice (details of the experiments are in section 5.1.2). Firstly, they are rendered in-situ and are augmented onto the drill axis for intuitive navigation and secondly they are rendered as an orthogonal projection to the viewing direction directly next to the region of interest for precise navigation (cf. figure 4.6(c)). This ensures that no information is lost due to the projective transformation and visualization and increases the confidence of the surgeons in their decisions and actions.

4.1.5 System Extensions to Enhance Depth Perception

Alternative approaches to provide a complete navigation and to improve the depth perception in video see-through head mounted display augmented reality were proposed within our research group by Bichlmeier et al., namely the concepts of virtual window [21], shadow [216], contextual mimesis [23], and the virtual mirror [22]. The virtual window was adopted from the original proposed one by Bajura et al. [12]. An especially promising technology is the virtual mirror concept, which facilitates the placement of a virtual mirror attached to an interaction device or a surgical device and thus enables to have an orthogonal/side view and control e.g. the insertion depth of instruments [22]. The concept was also successfully applied in 2D interfaces like augmented laparoscopy [165].

4.1 Hybrid Augmented Reality Navigation Interface

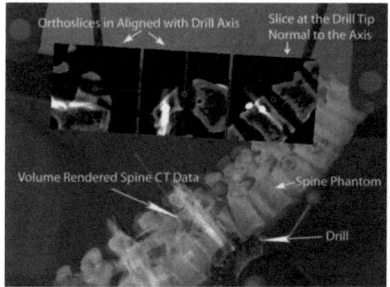
(a) Navigation and volume rendering.

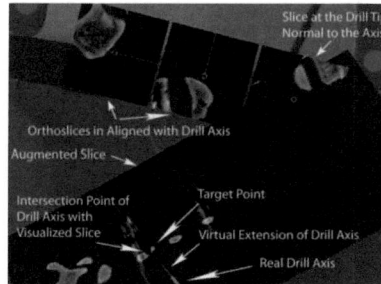
(b) With aligned slice view.

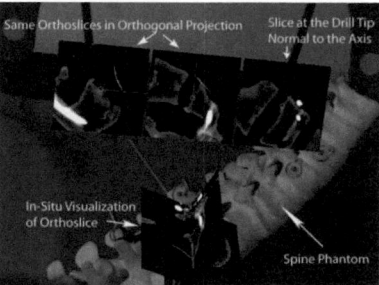
(c) With instrument aligned orthoslice view.

Figure 4.6: Different hybrid navigation modes combining in-situ and standard slice based navigation.

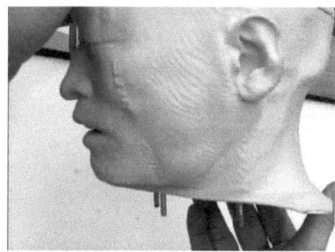
(a) Original video image.

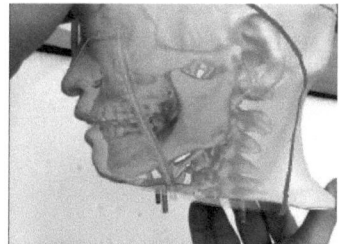
(b) Overlayed video image.

Figure 4.7: A focus and context visualization technique was adapted for the augmented reality system. The phantom is superimposed by a registered CT dataset. The images are rendered in real time with $\approx$ 30fps. Image courtesy of Oliver Kutter.

4.2 Camera Augmented Mobile C-Arm (CamC)

Another example for a navigation aid during percutaneous spinal interventions is the use of a C-arm system that is extended by a video camera. This chapter will explain the system setup in detail, discuss its limitations, and propose extensions for various applications. Experiments for determining the intrinsic system parameters and their results, as well as the results of simulated surgical procedures are presented in section 5.2. Additionally, the new system was compared to the state of the art procedure in a simulated vertebroplasty procedure. A theoretical model to compare different procedures based on the analysis of their common workflow phases and its application to the camera augmented mobile C-arm system are presented in section 5.3.

4.2.1 Related Work

The mobile C-arm is an essential tool in everyday routine trauma and orthopedics surgery. With increasing numbers of minimally invasive procedures the importance of CT and fluoroscopic guidance is still growing and so are the radiation doses [33, 231, 190, 234].

Considerable effort has been undertaken to improve the possibilities of CT and C-arm imaging especially in combination with external tracking systems to enable intraoperative navigation [110, 46, 147, 228, 229]. These procedures crucially change the current workflow and add additional technical complexity to the procedure. Most of these system require a fixation of a dynamic reference base (DRB), involve calibration and registration procedures, and introduce additional hardware components like an optical infrared tracking system.

Navigation systems based on CT or two and three dimensional C-arm data for spine surgery were introduced and discussed earlier (cf. section 3.3).

Augmented Imaging Devices: Most of the proposed in-situ visualization systems augment the view of the surgeon or an external camera with registered preoperative data. Several medical augmented reality systems were identified that directly augment intraoperatively acquired data onto the operation situs. These systems are also called augmented imaging devices. Stetten et al. [227] augment the real time image of an ultrasound transducer onto the target anatomy. Their system is called *sonic flashlight* and is based on a half silvered mirror and a flat panel miniature monitor mounted in a specific arrangement with respect to the ultrasound plane. Masamune et al. [146] proposed an arrangement of a half transparent mirror and a monitor rigidly attached to a CT scanner. With the correct relation between the mirror, monitor, and CT scanner, this system allows the visualization of one 2D CT slice in-situ. A similar technique was proposed for the in-situ visualization of a single MRI slice [60], however with different challenges to make it suitable for the MRI room. Leven et al. [135] augment the image of a laparoscopic ultrasound into the image of a laparoscope. Within their system they propose the system for the daVinci telemanipulator. A similar augmentation technique was applied by Feuerstein et al. [55] for freehand laparoscopic surgery based on intraoperatively acquired and three-dimensionally reconstructed C-arm data of contrasted liver vessels. Hayashibe et al. [85]

4.2 Camera Augmented Mobile C-Arm (CamC)

combined the registration free navigation approach with in-situ visualization. They use an intraoperatively tracked C-arm with reconstruction capabilities and a monitor that is mounted on a swivel arm providing volume rendered views from any arbitrary position.

Extended C-arm Device for Navigation: In [155] and [167] the early concepts for an extension of a mobile C-arm with an optical video camera attached to the housing of the gantry were proposed. Using a double mirror system and a one time calibration procedure during the construction of the system, the X-ray and optical images are aligned for all simultaneous acquisitions. If the patient and C-arm do not move, the X-ray images remain aligned with the video image. This makes the concept quite interesting for medical applications, particularly those which are currently based on permanent C-arm imaging. The concept was proposed for its use in controlling a needle placement procedure [155] and X-ray geometric calibration [156, 157]. With an early system setup only phantom studies were conducted.

The early concept of the system needed maturity and controlled studies before its clinical introduction. This was the objective of the performed accuracy analysis and of the phantom, and cadaver studies in close collaboration with a team of expert trauma surgeons (cf. section 5.2).

4.2.2 System Overview

The camera augmented mobile C-arm system extends a common intraoperative mobile C-arm by a color video camera (cf. section 4.2.2.1 and figure 4.8). A video camera and a double mirror system are constructed such that the X-ray source and the optical center of the video camera virtually coincide (cf. section 4.2.2.3). To enable an image overlay of the video and X-ray image in real time (cf. figure 4.15(a) and 4.15(b)) a homography has to be estimated that maps the X-ray image onto the video image (cf. section 4.2.2.3) taking the relative position of the X-ray detector implicitly into account (cf. section 4.2.2.2).

4.2.2.1 System Components

The C-arm used in the initial setup and the experiments is a Siremobile Iso-C 3D from Siemens Medical Solutions (Erlangen, Germany), a system that is used in our clinical laboratory for development as well as for phantom and cadaver studies. The video camera is a Flea from Point Grey Research Inc. (Vancouver, BC, Canada). The color camera includes a Sony 1/3" progressive scan CCD, with 1024x768 pixel resolution at a frame rate of 30FPS. The camera is connected via firewire (IEEE-1394) to the visualization computer, which is a standard PC extended by a Falcon framegrabber card from IDS Imaging Development System GmbH (Obersulm, Germany). The construction to mount the camera and the mirrors are custom made within our workshop. Without a mirror construction it is physically impossible to mount the video camera such that the X-ray source and the camera optical center virtually coincide. The mirror within the X-ray direction has to be X-ray transparent in order not to perturb the X-ray image quality. We also developed and adopted an interactive touchscreen based user interface for visualization and guidance (cf. section 4.2.2.4 and figure 4.16). This touchscreen enables direct

Two Novel Approaches to Image Guided Surgery

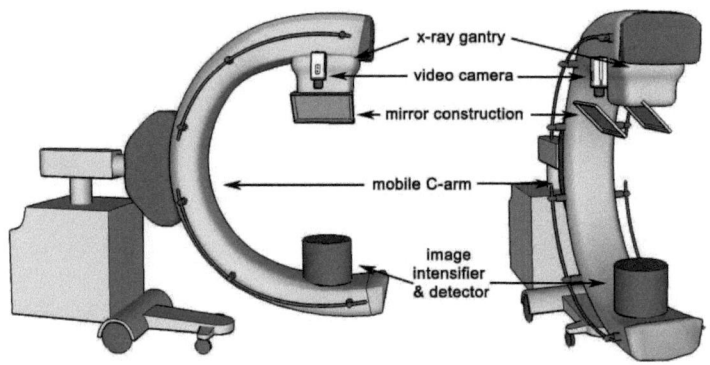

Figure 4.8: The camera augmented mobile C-arm system setup. The mobile C-arm is extended by an optical camera.

interaction with the imaging data presented on the monitor which is more intuitive to handle in an operative setup than a standard mouse/keyboard interaction.

4.2.2.2 System Calibration

Model of Optical Cameras Optical cameras, especially CCD cameras, are in general modeled as a pinhole camera. The camera model describes the mapping between 3D object points and their corresponding 2D image point using a central projection. The model in general is represented by an image plane and a camera center (cf. figure 4.10). The lens and the CCD sensor are in general in the same housing. This creates a fixed relationship between image plane and optical center. The projection geometry is commonly represented by $x = PX$ with $P \in \mathbb{R}^{3 \times 4}$ being the projection matrix, $X \in \mathbb{P}^3$ the object point in 3D, and $x \in \mathbb{P}^2$ its corresponding point in the image in projective space [83, 210].

Model of X-ray Imaging: The X-ray imaging is generally modeled as a point source with rays going through the object and imaged by the detector plane (cf. figure 4.11). X-ray geometry is often modeled using the same formulation as the optical video camera and with the same set of tools of projective geometry. However, in contrast to the optical camera model, the X-ray source and the detector plane are not rigidly constructed within one housing. Therefore, the X-ray source and the detector plane are loosely coupled, in fact they are mounted on opposite sides of the C-arm. [166] proposes a method based on definition of a virtual detector plane for compensation of the changes of relative position and orientation between X-ray source and detector plane. This method consists in imaging markers located on the X-ray housing near the X-ray source, so they are projected onto the borders of detector plane. The warping of these points to fixed virtual positions, often defined by a reference image, guarantees fixed intrinsic parameters, i.e. source-to-detector distance, image center, pixel size, and aspect ratio. The new 3D C-arms have

4.2 Camera Augmented Mobile C-Arm (CamC)

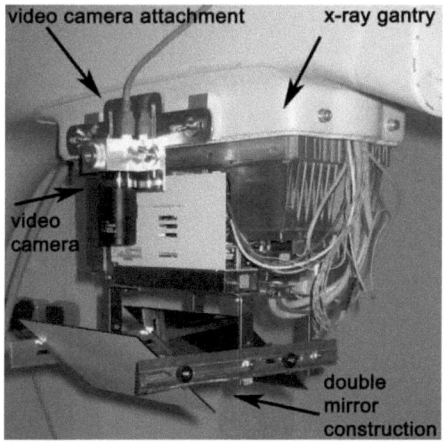

Figure 4.9: The video camera and the double mirror construction is physically attached such that it has the same optical center and optical axis than the X-ray source.

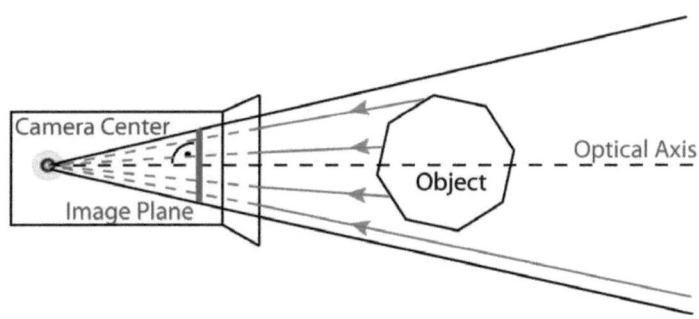

Figure 4.10: Geometric model of an optical camera.

69

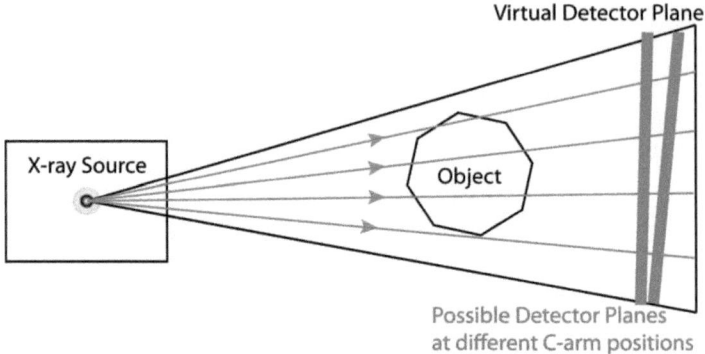

Figure 4.11: Geometric model of X-ray imaging.

more stable rotational movements and allow us to compute the required warping to the virtual detector during an off-line calibration procedure.

Three Step Calibration Procedure   The system calibration procedure is described and executed in three consecutive steps:

Step 1 - Distortion Correction: Both the images of the optical video camera and the X-ray system suffer from distortions. The optical camera distortion is estimated and corrected using standard computer vision methods. We use a non linear radial distortion model and pre-compute a look up table for fast distortion correction [242]. The radial lens distortion of the video camera is modeled by $X_{un} = D + X_{dist}$ with $X_{un} \in \mathbb{R}^2$ the undistorted point on the image, $X_{dist} \in \mathbb{R}^2$ the distorted one, and $D = X_{dist}(k_1 r^2 + k_2 r^4 + \ldots + k_i r^{2i})$ a polynomial function of the distortion coefficients k_i. The distortion coefficients are computed using well-known calibration techniques using a calibration pattern with known 3D geometry [86, 266][1]. The X-ray geometric distortion depends on the orientation of the mobile C-arm with regard to the earth's magnetic field, and thus is dependant on the angular, orbital, and wig-wag (room orientation) angle. For precise distortion correction, the C-arm has to be calibrated for every orientation. Look up tables provided by the vendor can however correct for the geometrical X-ray distortion for most common poses of the C-arm. For C-arms with solid state detectors instead of traditional image intensifiers, distortion is a minor problem and is often taken into account by system providers.

Step 2 - Alignment of X-ray Source and Camera Optical Center: The next step after the distortion correction consists of the positioning of the camera such that its optical center coincides with the X-ray source. This is achieved if a minimum of two undistorted rays, both optical and X-ray, pass through two pairs of markers located on two

---

[1] see Open Source Computer Vision Library http://www.intel.com/technology/computing/opencv/ for an exemplary implementation

4.2 Camera Augmented Mobile C-Arm (CamC)

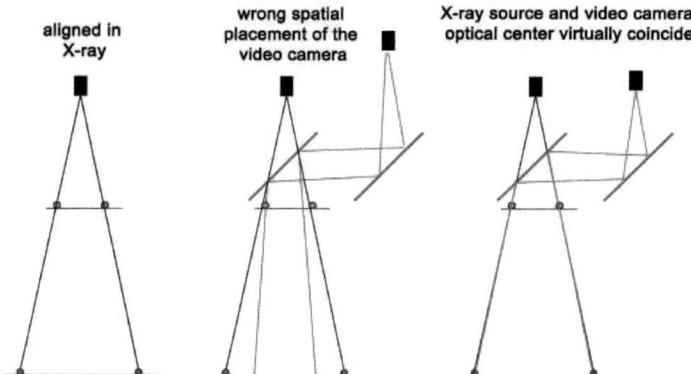

Figure 4.12: The video camera has to be attached such that it its optical camera center virtually coincides with the X-ray image source.

different planes (cf. figure 4.12). For one of the modalities, e.g. X-ray, this is simply done by positioning two markers on one plane and then positioning two others on the second plane such that their images coincide. This guarantees that the rays going through the corresponding markers on the two planes intersect at the projection center, e.g. the X-ray source. Due to parallax, the second modality will not view the pairs of markers aligned unless its projection center, e.g. camera center, is also at the intersection of the two rays defined by the two pairs of markers.

Step 3 - Homography Estimation for Image Overlay: After successful alignment of X-ray source and camera optical center, to enable an overlay of the images acquired by the X-ray device and video camera, a homography $H \in \mathbb{R}^{3 \times 3}$ is estimated. This homograpgh includes the translation on the image planes, the rotation around the normal of the image planes, and the pixel scaling between the video and X-ray image. This homography H is computed by a minimum of four corresponding points detected in the two images such that $p_{(v,i)} = H p_{(x,i)}$ with $p_{(v,i)}$ the 2D point in the video image and $p_{(x,i)}$ the corresponding point in the video image [83].

4.2.2.3 Implementation of System Calibration

The calibration procedure has to be performed only once during the initial attachment of the video camera and the double mirror construction to the gantry of the C-arm. It is valid as long as the optical camera and the mirror construction are not moved with respect to the X-ray gantry. We plan to incorporate the rigidly mounted construction into the housing of the C-arm gantry. After distortion correction (cf. section 4.2.2.2) the system calibration is performed using the following two steps:

Two Novel Approaches to Image Guided Surgery

Physical Placement of the Optical Camera and Mirror Construction The gantry mounted camera is physically placed such that its optical center is virtually aligned with the location of the X-ray source. This alignment is achieved by mounting the camera using a double mirror construction (cf. figure 4.9) with the support of a bi-planar calibration phantom (cf. figure 4.14). Our calibration phantom consists of two marker sets, each of them consisting of five markers that are arranged on a transparent plane and are visible both in X-ray and optically. The phantom is placed on the image intensifier of the C-arm. The markers on the far plane are rigidly attached spherical CT markers with 4mm diameter (CT-SPOTS, Beekley Corporation, Bristol, CT, USA). The markers on the near plane are aluminum rings that are moved such that they are pairwise overlaid with their spherical counterparts on the far plane in the X-ray image. In order to align all markers a series of X-ray images are acquired while moving the ring markers on the upper place (cf. figure 4.13). Once all markers are aligned in the X-ray image, the optical

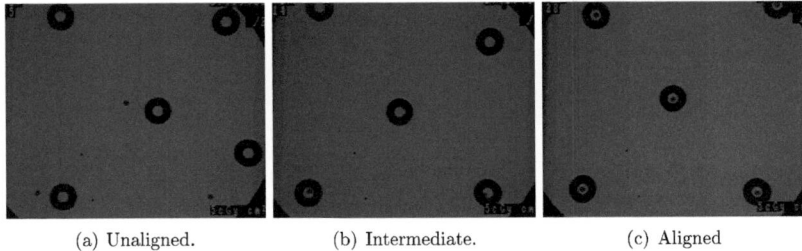

(a) Unaligned.   (b) Intermediate.   (c) Aligned

Figure 4.13: Sequence of X-ray images during the alignment of the markers on the biplanar calibration phantom.

video camera is attached such that all markers are also overlaid in the video image. The calibration phantom and the C-arm must not move until the final placement of the video camera is confirmed, i.e. the centers of all spherical markers are projected exactly in the center of the ring markers in the video image. Since this calibration step is a one time procedure during manufacturing of the device, a manual procedure for the research prototype is an acceptable solution. For a final assembly of the camera extended C-arm unit an algorithm enabling automatic extraction and visual servoing of the marker points and an apparatus for the placement in its optimal position could be realized with some additional engineering efforts.

Estimation of the Homography To superimpose the X-ray image onto the video image a homography $H_{I_x \to I_v} \in \mathbb{R}^{3\times 3}$ is computed, with I_v being the image of the video camera and I_x being the X-ray image. Any point p_x of the X-ray image can thus be wrapped to its corresponding point $p_{x \to v}$ on the video image I_v by $p_{x \to v} = H_{I_x \to I_v} p_x$. Within our application, we select a minimum of four corresponding points $p_{v,i}$ in the video image and $p_{x,i}$ in the X-ray image manually with the support of a subpixel accurate blob extraction algorithm. A semi-automatic establishment of the corresponding points

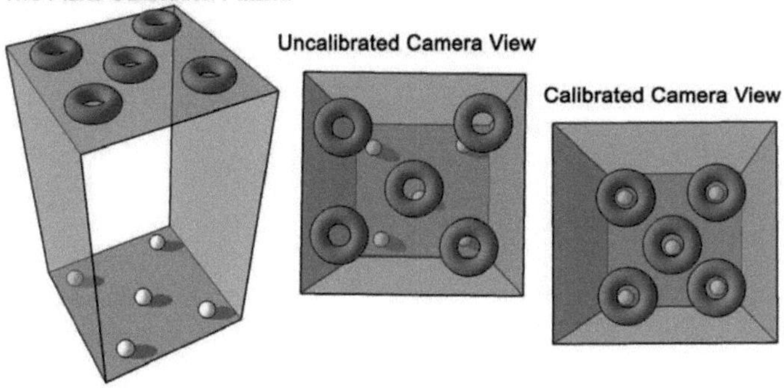

4.2 Camera Augmented Mobile C-Arm (CamC)

Two Plane Calibration Pattern

Uncalibrated Camera View

Calibrated Camera View

Figure 4.14: The bi-planar calibration phantom consists of X-ray and vision opaque markers. On the far plane at the bottom of the calibration phantom five spherical markers are rigidly attached. On the near plane there are five rings attached such that they can be moved and aligned with the spherical markers within the X-ray image.

is fine since the calibration has to be performed only once after the attachment of the video camera and the double mirror construction to the gantry and it is valid for a long time. The homography is computed by minimizing $argmin \sum_{i=1}^{n} \|p_{v,i} - H_{I_x \to I_v} p_{x,i}\|$ with $n > 3$ the number of corresponding points for the estimation of the homography. The resulting matrix $H_{I_x \to I_v}$ can be visually validated using the resulting image overlay (cf. figure 4.15(b)). As long as the video camera and the mirror construction is not moved with respect to the X-ray source, the calibration remains valid. The camera and mirror will be designed to remain inside the housing of the mobile C-arm and thus are not to be exposed to external forces which could modify the rigid arrangement. This means that the physical alignment and the estimation of the homography have to be performed only once during construction of the device. An evaluation of the calibration accuracy was performed and is discussed in section 5.2.

4.2.2.4 User Interface for Visualization and Navigation

The navigation software and user interface was developed in C++ based on our medical augmented reality framework (CAMPAR) [218] that is capable of synchronization of various input signals (e.g. image data). The basic user interface allows an overlay of the X-ray onto the video image (cf. figure 4.15(a) and 4.15(b)). Using standard mouse or touchscreen interaction a blending between fully opaque and fully transparent X-ray overlay is possible. Once the down-the-beam position of the C-arm is identified, i.e. the direction of insertion is exactly in the direction of the radiation beam, an entry point can

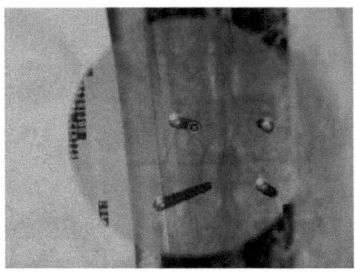 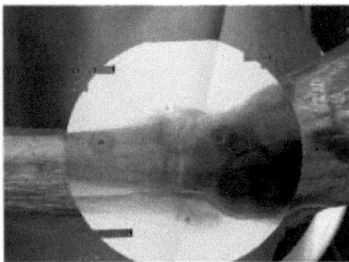

(a) Pedicle screw placement. (b) Foot augmentation.

Figure 4.15: Visualization of the image overlay system for spine and foot. The red crosshair defines one entry point for the ale or drill.

be identified in the X-ray image, which is directly visualized in the video image. Note that the down-the-beam positioning is an everyday task for a trauma surgeon and used in many applications under fluoroscopic control. The real time image overlay allows the surgeon to easily cut the skin for the instrumentation at the right location. It than provides the surgeon with direct feedback during the placement of the surgical instrument (e.g. guiding wire, awl, or drilling device) into the deep-seated target anatomy defined within the overlaid X-ray image (cf. figure 4.15(a) and 4.15(b)). This placement process does not involve any additional radiation for the patient and physician.

The image overlay is visualized on a standard monitor. This basic user interface was extended by a touchscreen monitor allowing easy interaction during the procedure. A modular implementation allows a fast integration of workflow adopted visualization [169] and control modules in order to extend system capabilities and customize the user interface for specific requirements for other applications (cf. figure 4.16).

4.2.3 Clinical Applications

There is a wide range of potential clinical applications for the camera augmented mobile C-arm system. For all procedures that are currently based on the intraoperative usage of mobile C-arms the new system can be seamlessly integrated into the clinical workflow, since no additional hardware has to be set up and no on-site calibration or registration has to be performed before and during the procedure.

4.2.3.1 Intraoperative Down-the-Beam Applications

One requirement for the smooth integration of the camera augmented mobile C-arm system into clinical workflow is to position the C-arm in the so called *down-the-beam* position, i.e. that the direction of insertion is exactly in the direction of the radiation beam. After positioning the C-arm, the entry point has to be defined in the X-ray image. The entry point has to match the axis of the instrument during the insertion and is thus based on the exact *down-the-beam* position of the C-arm and precise alignment of

4.2 Camera Augmented Mobile C-Arm (CamC)

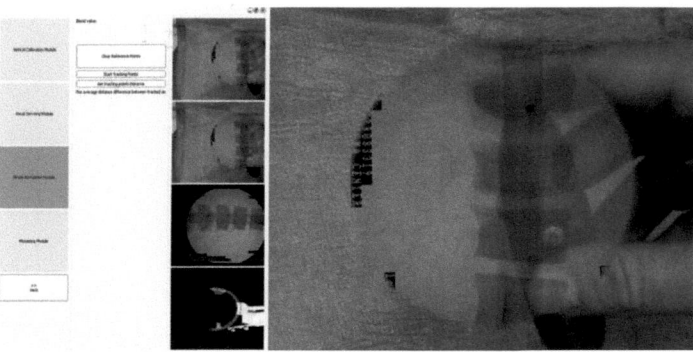

Figure 4.16: The user interface used for advanced visualization and guidance during the procedure. The interaction options (left) are implemented and visualized on a touchpad monitor and represent workflow, control and view modules (from left to right).

the instrument. The entry point is visualized also in the video image since the X-ray is co-registered with the video image by construction and one time calibration. Thus, the skin incision, the instrument tip alignment and the instrument axis alignment, i.e. to bring the instrument exactly into the *down-the-beam* position can be done only under video or fused video/X-ray control (cf. figure 4.17). Ideally the entire insertion process is performed using only one single X-ray image. To control the insertion depth additional lateral X-ray images are routinely acquired.

Interlocking of Intramedullary Nails The procedure for distal interlocking of intramedullary nails can be difficult and time consuming. Intramedullary nails are inserted into the bone marrow canal in the center of the long bones of the extremities (e.g. femur). The nail contains holes that are locked by screws from the outside. The challenge is to target these holes. Several guiding techniques and devices have been proposed to aid the guiding of the distal hole locking [259]. Many techniques, especially the free hand techniques without the use of targeting apparatus expose the patient, surgeon, and operation team to high doses of ionizing radiation. The camera augmented mobile C-arm following the usual positioning of the C-arm in the down-the-beam position, which is a routine procedure in C-arm based operations, can support the targeting of the distal holes and the locking procedure. In addition it is a considerable reduction of the radiation dose. The primary target is to move the C-arm in such a position that the interlocking hole is visualized. The fused image of X-ray and video enables a guidance aid for placing the interlocking nail drilling, as well as screw insertion (cf. figure 5.10). The depth can be controlled by direct haptic feedback. The surgeon can feel the difference between drilling in bone and soft tissue. A lateral X-ray image is not required during this procedure since the depth control is of no clinical importance in this application.

Two Novel Approaches to Image Guided Surgery

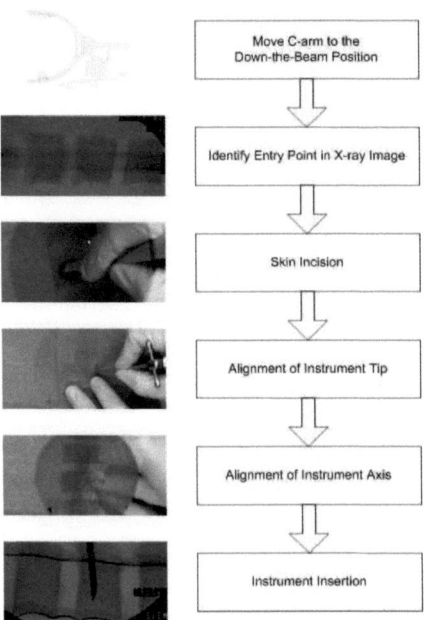

Figure 4.17: The typical medical workflow for an instrument insertion using the camera augmented mobile C-arm system.

4.2 Camera Augmented Mobile C-Arm (CamC)

Percutaneous Spinal Interventions (Pedicle Approach) The pedicle approach for minimally invasive spinal interventions remains a challenging task even after a decade of image guided surgery. This has lead to the development of a variety of computer aided techniques for dorsal pedicle interventions in the lumbar and thoracic spine [82, 147, 52]. Basic techniques use anatomical descriptions of the entry point and typical directions of the pedicle screws in conjunction with static X-ray control after instrumentation under intraoperative 2D fluoroscopic control. Advanced techniques use CT-Fluoro, CT, 2D, and 3D C-arm based navigation solutions.

The camera augmented mobile C-arm system can support the placement of the pedicle screws by means of an advanced visualization interface merging the real time video image and co-registered X-ray image. The only constraint for a proper use of the advanced visualization system is the down the beam positioning of the pedicle of interest. The direction for the pedicle screw must be aligned with the direction of the X-ray radiation. The guidance procedure is thus the alignment of the instrument (k-wire) at the entry point (aligning two degrees of freedom at the entry position) and then aligning the instrument within the viewing direction (aligning two degrees of freedom for the axis orientation). Commonly used surgical instruments need minor modifications in order to make the axis of the instrument better visible in the camera view.

4.2.3.2 Alternative Clinical Applications

Needle Guidance A possible application that is not exclusively dedicated to trauma and orthopedic surgery is the visual servoing for guidance of needle procedures as originally proposed for fluoroscopic imaging by Loser and Navab [142] and adopted by Mitschke et al. [155] for its usage with the camera augmented mobile C-arm system. The proposed system does not require the *down-the-beam* view of the C-arm. The system is based on a robotic visual servoing approach that moves a needle such that the projection of it in an arbitrary X-ray view is aligned with the deep-seated target. Based on visual servoing algorithms, the system recovers a plane including both the X-ray source and the deep-seated target. The needle remains aligned with the target in this X-ray view, while moving in this particular plane. The C-arm is then moved to a secondary position, ideally such at that the main X-ray direction is orthogonal to the plane recovered in the first iteration. The needle will be again aligned with the support of the visual servoing controlled robot in this secondary view. This results in a 3D alignment. The original process based on fluoroservoing required continuous fluoroscopic exposure. Using the camera augmented mobile C-arm system and video based visual servoing, the X-ray acquisition could theoretically be reduced to a minimum of two images. This is an interesting application for the CamC system, but this is not the focus application of our medical partners and therefore not evaluated further in this thesis.

X-ray Geometric Calibration: In addition to applications for instrument guidance, one clinical application is the improvement of X-ray geometric calibration by means of dynamic pose estimation using the attached video camera. For tomographic reconstruction, a sequence of images is captured during the orbital C-arm rotation around the object of interest. Every cone beam reconstruction of a C-arm [54] relies on the reproducibility of the C-arm motion, i.e. resulting in the same projection matrices for a given pose of the C-arm. This can however only be ensured for robotic or stationary C-arm systems. A dynamic calibration routine during the image acquisition process is required for a majority of mobile C-arms [163, 164]. In order to get the best estimation of the geometry X-ray opaque calibration phantoms could be used [120, 164, 199]. This is however impractical for on-line estimation of geometry since the markers of the calibration phantom have to be visible in every single frame and thus decrease the quality of the 3D reconstruction and occlude patient anatomy. There are two alternatives using optical imaging. The first is to use an external tracking system measuring the motion of markers attached to the C-arm, the second to attach one or more cameras to the C-arm itself. A previous study by Mitschke and Navab showed that an attached video camera outperforms the pose estimation of an external tracking system for 3D reconstruction [157]. Furthermore, it showed that the closer the optical center of the video camera is to the X-ray source, the more precise the estimation of the projection matrix is. Therefore, the camera augmented mobile C-arm system presents the theoretically optimal position of the attached optical camera for pose estimation. One should note that 3D reconstruction is only one particular application of dynamic calibration using the attached camera of the camera augmented mobile C-arm system. In general, since the attached camera has the same geometrical characteristics as the X-ray system, any application which needs the precise pose estimation for the X-ray device could make use of the optical camera. This could provide new technical solutions for many applications, which could be explored by the computer aided surgery community. In this thesis, I focus on the evaluation of well-defined clinical applications which are based on the down-the-beam positioning of the C-arm and are of interest to our medical partners.

Repositioning of the C-arm: The positioning and repositioning of the C-arm to image the region of interest is a delicate task in C-arm based diagnosis and therapy. This is to a large extent depending on the experience of the surgeon and often performed with the application of additional radiation dose for the identification of the desired target position of the C-arm with respect to the anatomy. The camera augmented mobile C-arm system can support this process by acquiring video images of the target position and then, knowing the model of the C-arm, guiding the C-arm back to this position only using the information of the video camera [171].

4.2.4 System Extension for Enabling Depth Control

The major limitation of the standard one camera augmented mobile C-arm system is that it only enables guidance for lateral instrument positioning, i.e. in the plane orthogonal to the optical axis of the camera. This means there is no control of the instrument insertion depth by the system, and lateral X-ray images need to be acquired. As an extension to the one camera system, a system was developed that is capable of depth control using only one additional X-ray image and a second video camera that is rigidly attached to the C-arm and orthogonal to the gantry [235]. An algorithm was implemented and integrated into

4.2 Camera Augmented Mobile C-Arm (CamC)

the system to track an instrument within the view of this orthogonally mounted camera. Using cross ratio, the position of the tip of the instrument is visualized in the laterally acquired X-ray image and thus allows guidance of the instrument in the anterior-posterior direction. In the following subsections the system setup and system calibration for the two camera solution as well as its benefit for clinical applications and initial feasibility tests are described.

4.2.4.1 System Setup

The two camera solution extends the same C-arm that was used for the one camera augmented mobile C-arm system (cf. section 4.2.2.1), the Iso3D C-arm (Siemens Medical, Erlangen, Germany). Both cameras attached are Flea video color cameras (Point Grey Research Inc., Vancouver, BC, Canada) (see figure 4.18). The first camera is mounted at the gantry exactly at the same position and with the same method as described earlier for the one camera augmented mobile C-arm solution (cf. section 4.2.2.3). The second camera is mounted orthogonally to the gantry such that its image is aligned with the X-ray image after a 90 degrees orbital rotation of the C-arm (see figure 4.18). The same standard PC was used. The visualization and navigation software was extended to support the second camera image overlay and tool tracking.

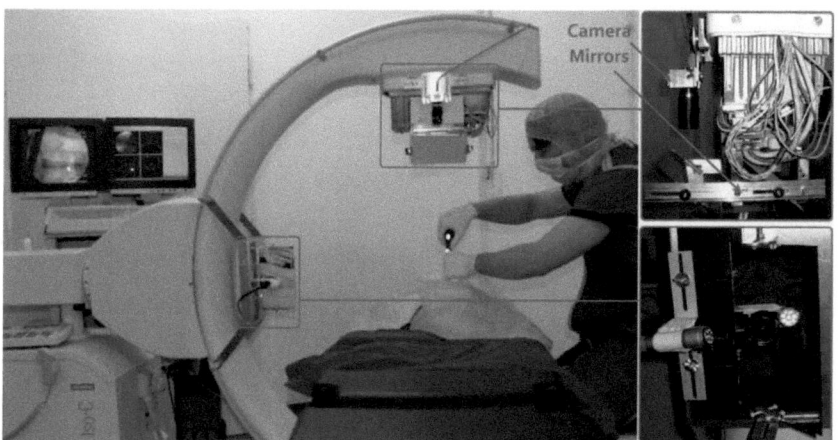

Figure 4.18: The C-arm with two attached video cameras. The first camera is attached to the gantry with a double mirror construction. The second camera is attached in an orthogonal direction with a single mirror construction. The C-arm is positioned in the 0 degree orbital position.

System Calibration for the Orthogonally Mounted Video Camera The calibration method for the orthogonally mounted camera is similar to the method proposed for

Two Novel Approaches to Image Guided Surgery

the gantry mounted camera (cf. section 4.2.2.3). Again, the calibration process is composed of two consecutive steps. In the first step the camera is physically attached such that the optical center and axis virtually coincide with the X-ray imaging system at a particular C-arm position e.g. in 90 degree orbital rotation for the orthogonally mounted camera. The second step is to compute the homography to align the video image with the X-ray image acquired after this orbital rotation. Prior to this two step procedure the image of the orthogonally mounted camera is undistorted with the same method as described in section 4.2.2.2 for the gantry mounted camera.

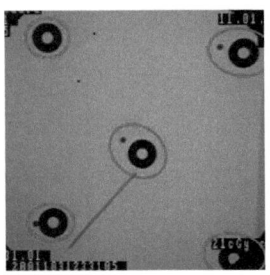 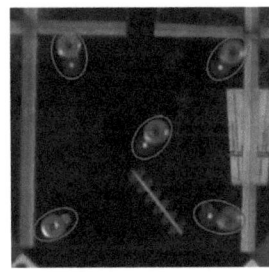 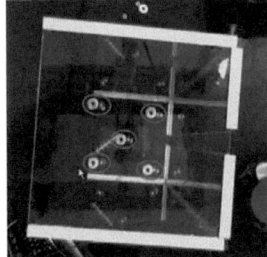

(a) X-ray with misaligned markers. (b) Camera 1 with misaligned markers. (c) Camera 2 with misaligned markers.

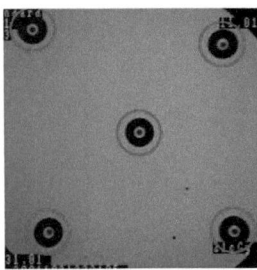 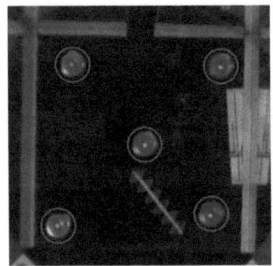 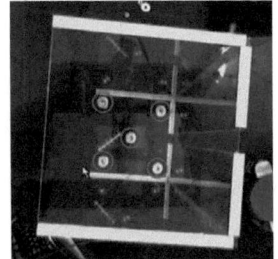

(d) X-ray with aligned markers. (e) Camera 1 with aligned markers. (f) Camera 2 with aligned markers.

Figure 4.19: The calibration phantom in the different imaging systems.

Notation: Since we have X-ray and video images at different positions of the C-arm, superscript 0 denotes images acquired at a 0 degree orbital rotation (i.e. the standard down-the-beam position of the C-arm as illustrated in figure 4.18) and superscript 90 denotes images acquired by the C-arm after an orbital rotation around 90 degrees. Furthermore subscript x is used for X-ray images, g for images of the gantry mounted camera, and o for images of the orthogonal mounted camera.

X-ray to Orthogonally Mounted Camera Calibration: We constrained the attachment of the second camera to be about orthogonal to the C-arm gantry. An orthogonal attachment provides best results for the depth navigation, assuming the instruments to always be used down-the-beam as required in the single camera navigation system (cf. section 4.2.3). The physical attachment and calibration of the second camera at alternative positions is also possible with the same calibration procedure described in this paragraph.

To acquire an X-ray image at 90 degrees rotation I_x^{90}, corresponding to the image of the orthogonally mounted video camera before the rotation I_o^0, we have to ensure that the camera center of the orthogonally mounted video camera before the rotation coincides with the X-ray source after the orbital rotation around 90 degrees. Since the gantry mounted camera is already physically aligned with the X-ray device (cf. section 4.2.2.2), the problem can be reduced to aligning the optical center of the gantry mounted camera before the rotation and the optical center of the orthogonally mounted camera after the 90 degrees rotation. This alignment is achieved with the same bi-planar calibration pattern (cf. figure 4.14) that is used for the positioning of the gantry mounted camera. A set of markers is placed on each plane such that subsets of two markers, one marker on each plane, are aligned in one ray of the image of the gantry mounted camera I_g^0 at the initial, 0 degree position of the C-arm (cf. figure 4.19(e)). In the next step, the C-arm is rotated by -90 degrees in orbital direction (cf. figure 4.19(c)). The orthogonally mounted camera is attached such that all marker tuples from the calibration pattern are lined up in image I_o^{-90} (cf. figure 4.19(f)). Note that this calibration has to be performed only once during the construction of the system. The calibration is valid until external force perturbs the spatial relationship between X-ray source and mounted video cameras.

For a proper alignment of the lateral X-ray image I_x^{90} after 90 degree rotation in orbital direction and the image I_o^0 of the orthogonally mounted camera with 0 degree rotation, two homographies remain to be computed. A first homography $H_{I_g^{90} \leftarrow I_x^{90}}$ that maps the X-ray image I_x^{90} to the gantry mounted image in 90 degrees orbital rotation I_g^{90} and a second homography $H_{I_o^0 \leftarrow I_g^{90}}$ mapping the image of the gantry mounted camera I_g^{90} to the image of the orthogonal mounted camera at 0 degree orbital rotation I_o^0. The final homography used to map the X-ray image I_x^{90} taken at 90 degree orbital rotation onto the orthogonally mounted camera image I_o^0 at 0 degree rotation $H_{I_o^0 \leftarrow I_x^{90}} = H_{I_o^0 \leftarrow I_g^{90}} \cdot H_{I_g^{90} \leftarrow I_x^{90}}$ is a combination of the two homographies computed earlier. Both homographies are computed using corresponding points in the images the same way as in section 4.2.2.3 for the one camera augmented mobile C-arm solution.

Instrument Tracking The surgical tool is extended by three collinear markers on the instrument axis. We use retro-reflective circular markers that are illuminated by an additional light source attached to the orthogonally mounted camera. This setup results in the markers being seen by the orthogonal camera as bright ellipses, which can be easily and robustly detected in the image by basic thresholding and region growing algorithms. From the binary image created by thresholding all contours are extracted using the Intel OpenCV library. In a post-processing step we filter those contours with a low compactness value and the ones that are smaller than an area threshold (the used default values are 0.6 for compactness and 50 pixels as area threshold). For all contours being retained by the

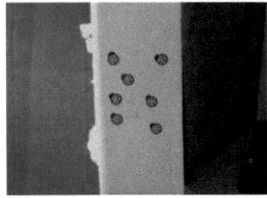 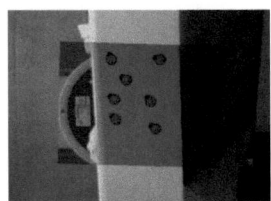 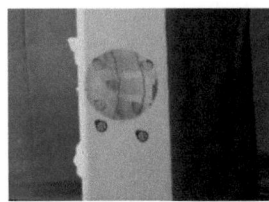

(a) Image of the orthogonally mounted camera.
(b) Gantry mounted camera image overlay after applying $H_{I_o^0 \leftarrow I_g^{90}}$.
(c) X-ray image overlay after applying $H_{I_o^0 \leftarrow I_x^{90}}$.

Figure 4.20: Estimation of the homographies that are used to superimpose the image of the gantry mounted video camera I_g^{90} and the X-ray image I_x^{90} after rotation onto the image of the orthogonally mounted camera I_o^0.

filtering routine, the centroids are computed with sub-pixel accuracy based on grayscale image moments. Finally the three detected contours are used for an optimal least squares line fitting, assuming the most significant detected ones to be the markers of the tool.

Having the three collinear markers detected in the 2D image plane and given the 3D geometry of our instrument, i.e. the position of the distal end of the instrument with respect to the three markers, we are able to compute the tip of the instrument in the image. For the estimation of the tip in the image we use the constraint that the cross-ratio is invariant in projective transformations [210].

$$cross = \frac{d_{12}d_{23}}{d_{13}d_{24}} = \frac{\Delta x_{12} \Delta x_{23}}{\Delta x_{13} \Delta x_{24}} = \frac{\Delta y_{12} \Delta y_{23}}{\Delta y_{13} \Delta y_{24}} \quad (4.3)$$

Here, d_{ij} are the distances in three dimensions between the markers i and j, or between a marker and the tool tip. Investigating the distances in the image in x- and y-direction separately gives us Δx_{ij} and Δy_{ij}, where $\Delta x_{24} = |x_2 - x_4|$ and $\Delta y_{24} = |y_2 - y_4|$ contain the unknown coordinates x_4 and y_4 of the instrument tip in the image. Since the X-ray image I_x^{90} is by construction co-registered with the video image I_o^0 of the orthogonally mounted camera by $H_{I_o^0 \leftarrow I_x^{90}}$, we can estimate the position of the tip in the X-ray image I_x^{90} taken at 90 degrees rotation (cf. figure 4.22(c)).

4.2.4.2 Navigation and Surgical Workflow

The navigation does not require any further online calibration or registration procedure during the surgery. The previously described calibration routine has to be performed only once while the system is built and is valid as long as the cameras do not move with respect to the C-arm gantry.

The workflow of the two camera augmented mobile C-arm system can be described in eight consecutive steps (cf. figure 4.21):

1. The C-arm is placed in the initial, down-the-beam position that means the direction of the X-rays are aligned with the direction of insertion of the instrument.

4.2 Camera Augmented Mobile C-Arm (CamC)

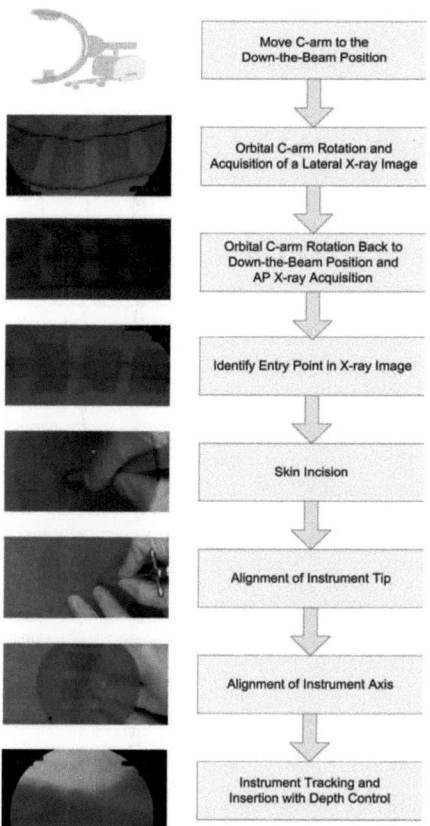

Figure 4.21: The typical surgical workflow for an instrument insertion using the two camera augmented mobile C-arm system that enables lateral instrument positioning and depth control.

2. The C-arm is rotated exactly 90 degrees in orbital direction. To support this 90 degrees rotation a visual guidance was implemented. An image I_o^0 of the orthogonally mounted camera is captured before the rotation starts. The captured image I_o^0 is overlaid with a live video image during the rotation of the gantry mounted camera $I_g^0 \ldots I_g^{90}$ that is transformed by homography $H_{I_o^0 \leftarrow I_g^{90}}$ to visually guide the 90 degrees rotation process. This will ensure that the gantry mounted camera has the same position and orientation as the second camera had before the 90 degrees rotation. Any subsequently acquired and stored lateral X-ray image I_x^{90} corresponds to the image of the gantry mounted camera at 90 degrees orbital rotation I_g^{90} as well

as to the captured image of the orthogonal camera I_o^0 before the rotation and the live image of the orthogonally mounted camera after rotating back exactly 90 degrees.

3. The C-arm is rotated back to the initial, down-the-beam position. The rotation back is guided using combined X-ray and optical markers attached to the side of our surgical object that are visible in the X-ray image I_x^{90} and the image I_o^0 of the orthogonal camera. Thus the X-ray image I_x^{90} we have taken at the 90 degrees C-arm position perfectly corresponds to the image of the orthogonally mounted camera with 0 degree orbital rotation I_o^0 after applying the pre-computed homography $H_{I_o^0 \leftarrow I_x^{90}}$. In the initial down-the-beam position a second X-ray image I_x^0, an anterio-posterior (AP) image, is acquired that is directly overlaid onto the image gantry mounted camera I_g^0 in this C-arm position.

4. The entry point for instrument insertion is defined based on the anterior-posterior X-ray image I_x^0.

5. The skin incision is performed using the image overlay of the anterior-posterior X-ray image I_x^0 and the image of the gantry mounted camera I_g^0. A valid overlay is facilitated by the pre-computed homography $H_{I_g^0 \leftarrow I_x^0}$ (cf. figure 4.22(a)).

6. The tool is positioned in lateral direction using image overlay of the anterior-posterior X-ray image I_x^0 and the image of the gantry mounted camera I_g^0.

7. The tool is aligned in the down-the-beam direction using the image overlay of the anterior-posterior X-ray image I_x^0 and the image of the gantry mounted camera I_g^0. The extention of the tool is projected into the lateral X-ray image I_x^{90} and can be used to correct the alignment of the instrument before insertion, especially in craniocaudal direction.

8. The tool is inserted using both image overlay views, the overlay of the gantry mounted camera image I_g^0 with the anterior-posterior X-ray image I_x^0 for the initial position and orientation of the tool and the orthogonally mounted camera image I_o^0 overlaid by the laterally acquired X-ray image I_x^{90} (cf. figure 4.22) . This is combined with tool tracking for the control of the insertion depth and additional control in craniocaudal direction (cf. figure 4.22(c)).

4.2.4.3 Preclinical Experiments with the Two Camera Solution

The feasibility of the system was tested on a spine phantom. We used a tracked awl, a pedicle probe, and a T-handle to place pedicle screws. Using an orthogonal control X-ray image we could visually verify the accuracy of the depth navigation (cf. figure 4.2.4.3).

In a cadaver experiment we placed eight pedicle screws (Universal Spine System USS, Synthes, Umkirch) with a diameter of 6.2 mm in four vertebrae of the thoracic and lumbar spine (T12, L1, L2, and L3). The surgical procedure was carried out in three steps using a pedicle awl to open the cortical bone, a pedicle probe to penetrate the pedicle, and a T-handle for screw implantation. For the guided procedure both augmented views, the

4.2 Camera Augmented Mobile C-Arm (CamC)

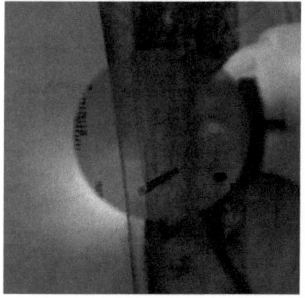 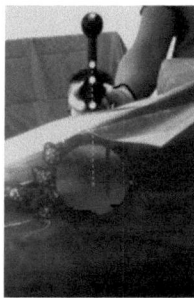 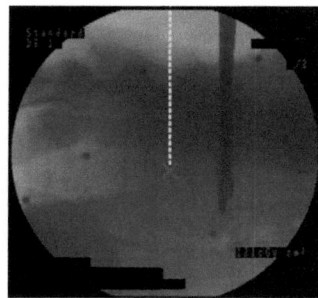

(a) Image overlay of the gantry mounted camera I_g^0 for lateral positioning.

(b) Image overlay of the orthogonally mounted camera I_o^0 for insertion depth estimation.

(c) Superimposition of the insertion depth estimation onto the lateral X-ray image I_x^{90}.

Figure 4.22: The navigation interface includes the lateral positioning of the instrument and the insertion depth estimation.

one for lateral instrument positioning (see figure 4.23(a)) and the one for depth control (see figure 4.23(b)), were used simultaneously presented on two monitors. After aligning the C-arm imaging system in the down-the-beam position for the instrumentation, the acquisition of only two X-ray images was sufficient for each of the eight pedicle screws. This is a considerable reduction of radiation compared to the standard procedure, which is performed under fluoroscopy control.

The accuracy of the pedicle screw placement was verified by a postinterventional CT-scan ((cf. figure 4.24(a) and 4.24(b))) using a clinical scale proposed by Arand et al. [6]. Five pedicle screws were classified by a medical expert to be in group A, i.e. central screw position without perforation. The other three screws were classified to be in group B, i.e. lateral screw perforation within thread diameter. For none of the eight pedicle screws a medial perforation in direction of the spinal canal occurred.

One critical remark is that neither the surgical object nor the C-arm system is supposed to move during the navigated procedure. Attached markers that are visible in video and X-ray images in combination with an automatic marker detection can notify the surgeon in case of C-arm system or patient movement. This will result in the acquisition of two additional X-ray images in 90 degrees (I_x^{90}) and 0 degree (I_x^{90}) position. First cadaver experiments demonstrated that the new system can be easily integrated into the clinical workflow while considerably reducing the radiation dose compared to the current clinical routine. The observed accuracy during the experiments is clinically acceptable.

4.2.5 System Extension for Visual Servoing

The positioning and repositioning of a C-arm to image the region of interest is a challenging task in C-arm based diagnosis and therapy. The positioning is to a large extent based on the experience and skill of the surgeon and often applies extra radiation dose for

Two Novel Approaches to Image Guided Surgery

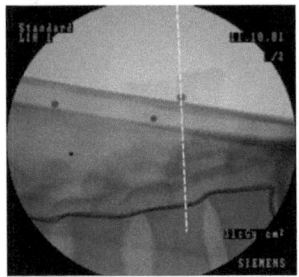 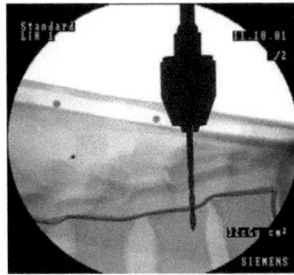

(a) Tracked instrument projected in lateral X-ray image I_x^{90}. (b) Real instrument in the lateral control X-ray image I_x^{90}.

Figure 4.23: Visual validation of the tracked tool projected in the lateral X-ray image I_x^{90} and a lateral control X-ray image with the inserted tool.

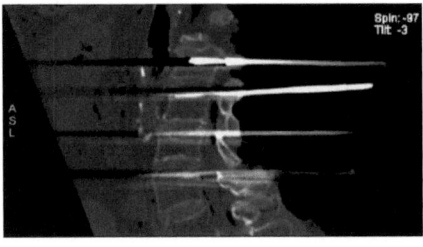 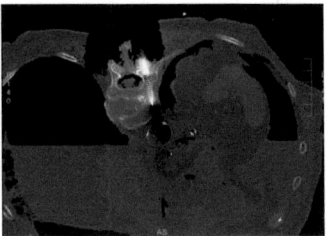

(a) Sagittal plane. (b) Transversal plane.

Figure 4.24: Evaluation with postinterventional CT data of the cadaver study. The shown screws have a good insertion depth and show a good placement in craniocaudal direction.

the placement of the C-arm in the desired target position. The camera augmented mobile C-arm can support the process in positioning the C-arm such that it images the region of interest. An alternative system is based on the projection of a laser cross hair onto the surface of the patient and manual marking of the position of the laser on the patient's skin before moving the C-arm. This is however only valid if the surface does not deform.

The camera augmented mobile C-arm system can support the process of positioning and repositioning the mobile C-arm by acquiring a video image of the target position and then knowing the model the C-arm, its joints and configuration, being able to guide the C-arm back to this position only using the information extracted from the attached video camera [171]. The work is in an early stage and was implemented and tested on rigid marker configurations. Its extension to deformable marker models and the validity of the visual servoing under real conditions has to be investigated.

4.2 Camera Augmented Mobile C-Arm (CamC)

4.2.5.1 System Configuration for Visual Servoing

Video visible markers are placed within the surgical scene such that they are visible in the reference position, i.e. the position the C-arm has to be guided to, and start position, i.e. the position of the C-arm from where it is guided to the reference position. Markers with a high contrast compared to the surgical scene are used to easily and robustly extract them within the video image (cf. figure 4.25 for the used phantom).

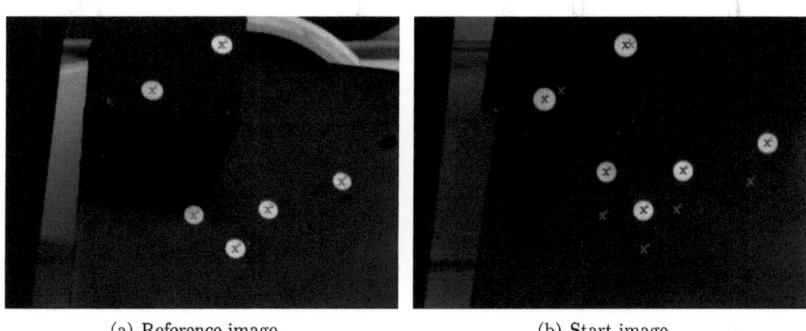

(a) Reference image. (b) Start image.

Figure 4.25: Reference and start video image for the visual servoing. The red crosses indicate the extracted centroids in the target image (also projected into the start image) and the blue crosses indicate the extracted and tracked centroids in the start and current image.

The procedure to apply the visual servoing for the camera augmented mobile C-arm system contains five steps:

1. **Capture Reference Image:** An image at the reference position is captured before (re)moving the C-arm. The centroids of the markers are extracted.

2. **Initializing of Guidance:** The C-arm is placed in the start position with zero joint configuration. All markers need to be visible in the image of the video camera at the start position.

3. **Track Markers:** The marker centroids in the current image are extracted and tracked while the C-arm is moved.

4. **Estimate C-arm Motion:** The motion of the C-arm is estimated within the coordinate system of the C-arm. The estimation is performed using independently a 2D and 3D algorithm. Both are based on the marker positions in the current image, the marker positions in the reference image, and a model of the C-arm.

5. **Convergence:** Step 4 is repeated until the root mean square error of the markers in the reference and current image is below a defined threshold.

Joint no.	Type	Unit	C-arm motion
1	prismatic	m	height
2	revolute	rad	wigwag
3	prismatic	m	length
4	revolute	rad	angular
5	revolute	rad	orbital

Table 4.1: C-arm joints overview

Joint no.	a (Trans$_x$)	d (Trans$_z$)	α (Rot$_x$)	ϕ (Rot$_z$)
1	0	height	0	0
2	0	0	$-\pi/2$	wigwag
3	0	length	0	$-\pi/2$
4	0	1.5	$\pi/2$	angular
5	0.7	0	0	orbital
6	0	0	$\pi/2$	$-\pi/2$

Table 4.2: The used Denavit-Hartenberg parameters to model the C-arm.

4.2.5.2 C-arm Kinematics

The forward kinematics of the C-arm is modeled using the Denavit-Hartenberg rules for the five joints (cf. table 4.1). These define the position of the end effector, i.e. the C-arm gantry, dependent on the joint values.

T^i_{i+1} is the coordinate transformation from the coordinate frame of joint i to joint $i+1$. The final position of the C-arm gantry (end effector) is a concatenation of all joint transformations:

$$\mathcal{F}_{ee} = T^0_1 T^1_2 T^2_3 T^3_4 T^4_5 T^5_6 \quad (4.4)$$

Table 4.2 shows the details of the used parameters. An additional fixed sixth transformation takes into account the rotation between the coordinate system of the fifth joint and the coordinate system of the camera.

4.2.5.3 Mathematical Problem Statement

Given is a set of n marker points $P_1, ... P_n \in \mathbb{R}^3$ fixed in three dimensional space.

A two dimensional projection of these points is made at reference position $\mathcal{F}^*$ and at start position $\mathcal{F}$. The projected points in the image at the reference position $\mathcal{F}^*$ are $S_{\mathcal{F}^*} = (S^*_1, \ldots S^*_n)$, $S^*_{1...n} \in \mathbb{R}^2$ and at the start position $\mathcal{F}$ they are $S_{\mathcal{F}} = (S_1, \ldots S_n)$, $S_{1...n} \in \mathbb{R}^2$. The correspondences between the extracted points $S_i \leftrightarrow S^*_i, i \in \{1, \ldots n\}$ are known.

The start position $\mathcal{F}$ denotes the "zero" joint configuration i.e. $q = (0,0,0,0,0)^T$. $\mathcal{F}^*$ is the position of the C-arm gantry at the unknown joint configuration $q^* = (q^*_1, \ldots q^*_5)^T$.

The aim of the visual servoing algorithm is to find a sequence of m joint configurations $q_k, k \in 1, \ldots m$ with $q_1 = q$ and $q_m = q^*$ where consecutive joint configurations q_k and q_{k+1} differ only in one joint manipulation. The aim is to minimize the number of iterations m.

4.2 Camera Augmented Mobile C-Arm (CamC)

At the position $\mathcal{F}_k$ (defined by joint configuration q_k) the projections $S_{\mathcal{F}_k}$ of the points $P_1, \ldots P_n$ are known and used to estimate the next joint motion. The final reference position $\mathcal{F}^*$ with joint configuration q^* is reached once $S_{\mathcal{F}_k}$ approaches $S_{\mathcal{F}^*}$, which means that the projections on the images $S_m \approx S_{\mathcal{F}^*}$ and the C-arm gantry position $\mathcal{F}_m \approx \mathcal{F}^*$ are almost identical.

It is also assumed that the points $P_1, \ldots P_n$ are in such a configuration so that if $S_{\mathcal{G}} = S_{\mathcal{F}^*}$ it follows that $\mathcal{G} = \mathcal{F}^*$. This means that the marker configuration must designed such that it leads to an unambiguous relation between a set of projected points $S_{\mathcal{G}}$ and the pose of the C-arm gantry $\mathcal{G}$. West et al. [258] state that near-collinear marker configurations should be avoided. Bruckstein et al. [39] prove the optimum configuration under weak perspective projection to be "when the points form concentric complete regular polyhedra". Liu et al. [138] use genetic algorithms to improve marker configurations for pose estimation.

4.2.5.4 Two Dimensional Visual Servoing Algorithm

One possible solution uses image based visual servoing where the extracted marker centroids of reference and starting image are used to control the C-arm motion [223]. This was implemented and tested for the camera augmented mobile C-arm [171]. An error function is defined based on the difference in image coordinates of the marker centroids at the starting (current) position and the reference position. With a control law this error can be directly mapped to a C-arm motion.

Manipulator Jacobian: The Cartesian velocity v_{ee} of the end effector is described by its linear and angular velocity.

$$v_{ee} = (\gamma_x, \gamma_y, \gamma_z, \omega_x, \omega_y, \omega_z)^T \tag{4.5}$$

v_{ee} is dependent on the velocities $\dot{q}_i$ of the single joints.

$$\dot{q} = (\dot{q}_1, \dot{q}_2, \dot{q}_3, \dot{q}_4, \dot{q}_5))^T \tag{4.6}$$

The relationship between joint velocity and C-arm gantry velocity can be given in a linear equation

$$v_{ee} = J_q \dot{q}. \tag{4.7}$$

$J_q \in \mathbb{R}^{6 \times 5}$ is the so called *manipulator Jacobian*. It is the Jacobian matrix that contains the partial derivates of the position of the C-arm with respect to the joint values. Here the manipulator Jacobian is always given in the base coordinate system of the C-arm. The Jacobian depends on the current joint configuration. Thus, we always assume a zero joint position at the beginning of the 2D visual servoing algorithm ($q_1 = q = (0,0,0,0,0)^T$). Each column of the Jacobian corresponds to one of the five joints of the C-arm joint.

Interaction Matrix for Point Features: A projection $S_{\mathcal{F}_{i-1}} = \left(S_1^{(i-1)}, \ldots S_n^{(i-1)}\right)$ of the points $P_1, \ldots P_n$ is made at position $\mathcal{F}_{i-1}$. Another projection $S_{\mathcal{F}_i}$ is made at position $\mathcal{F}_i \neq \mathcal{F}_{i-1}$. The difference of the projected points $\Delta S_i = S_{\mathcal{F}_i} - S_{\mathcal{F}_{i-1}}$ is the velocity of the projected points. If the timestep between the two projections is defined to be 1 second, the difference is the velocity of the points at time i:

$$\dot{S}_{\mathcal{F}_i} = S_{\mathcal{F}_i} - S_{\mathcal{F}_{i-1}} \tag{4.8}$$

The interaction matrix $L_i \in \mathbb{R}^{2 \times 6}$ relates the velocity of the C-arm gantry v_{ee} to the velocity of one projected point P_i. L_i depends on an estimated depth z of the point P_i along the optical axis of the projection and the projected points $S_i = (x/z, y/z)^T = (s_x, s_y)^T$.

In order to use all projected points in the images, the complete interaction matrix $L \in \mathbb{R}^{2n \times 6}$ is built for all n points:

$$\begin{pmatrix} \dot{S}_1 \\ \vdots \\ \dot{S}_n \end{pmatrix} = \begin{pmatrix} L_1 \\ \vdots \\ L_n \end{pmatrix} v_{ee} = L v_{ee} \tag{4.9}$$

Control Law: A control law gives rules how to adjust a system to minimize a given cost function. This is mostly done in a closed loop circuit, where the desired value is continuously compared with the actual value.

In this case, the cost function is the error $e(t) = S(t) - S^*$ of the projected coordinates at a certain time t.

$$\dot{e}(t) = \frac{d}{dt}(S(t) - S^*) = \dot{S}(t) = L v_{ee}. \tag{4.10}$$

In order to solve for v_{ee}, we use the approximated pseudo-inverse of L computed with $L^+ \approx \left(\hat{L}^T \hat{L}\right)^{-1} \hat{L}$.

The joint updates can be computed with the pseudo-inverse of the manipulator Jacobian by

$$\dot{q} = J_q^+ v_{ee} \tag{4.11}$$

In the discrete case $\dot{q}$ is written as $\Delta q_i = q_{i+1} - q_i$ and

$$\Delta q = -\lambda J_{q_i}^+ \hat{L}^+ (S_i - S^*). \tag{4.12}$$

A single joint has to be selected because only one joint can be moved at a time. Experimental results showed that the joint with the maximum absolute joint difference leads to the fastest convergence of the algorithm. In order to be able to compare revolute joints with prismatic joints, the revolute joint values are multiplied by their distance to the next joint. For the model of the C-arm this results in the weights $w = (1, 1.5, 1, 0.7, 0.7)^T$ and thus the weighted joint increments $\Delta q^{(w)} = \Delta q \cdot w$.

The fact, that only one joint can be moved in each iteration makes the convergance of the system slower. Since the algorithms depends on a known current joint configuration it is required to move the joint exactly the magnitude proposed by the algorithm, since it is not possible to access the joint configuration by the C-arm system directly. This can

4.2 Camera Augmented Mobile C-Arm (CamC)

also cause that the algorithm does not converge towards the reference position and should be subject to more detailed investigations.

Therefore in our experiments we only moved the joint with the maximum of the absolute joint values at a time, and thus the required sequence of joint configurations q_k is defined by the system.

4.2.5.5 Three Dimensional Visual Servoing Algorithm

If the $3D$ geometry of the points $P_1, ... P_n \in \mathbb{R}^3$ is known within their local object coordinate system, the relative position between the points and the camera can be recovered (for specific marker configurations). First the points are registered in the C-arm base coordinate system. This means that the local object coordinates are transformed into the C-arm base coordinates. After that, pose estimation from the attached camera gives the position of the C-arm gantry in C-arm base coordinates since the camera optical center and X-ray source coincide by construction. This is done for both C-arm positions, the current position and the reference position. Inverse kinematics gives the joint configuration of the C-arm gantry pose for both positions. From the difference between the two configurations the required joint movement can be directly extracted.

For the pose estimation from corresponding 2D projections and 3D points the approach of Hager et al. [143] is used. This approach minimized the object space error.

4.2.5.6 Evaluation of the Visual Servoing Algorithms

The $2D$ and $3D$ algorithms were implemented into our existing software framework in C++. Several experiments were conducted to show the performance of the algorithms. For a ground truth measurement of the C-arm gantry repositioning accuracy, the C-arm gantry was extended by marker target of an external optical tracking device (cf. section 1.2.3.1). A calibration of the tracking target coordinate system with the camera coordinate system allows us to get the position $\mathcal{F}_T$ of the X-ray source with high accuracy. It furthermore facilitates a comparison between the reference position $\mathcal{F}_T^*$ and the position $\mathcal{F}_{T,i}$ after i iterations. It provides a measurement criterion for the quality of the recovered C-arm gantry pose in base coordinates.

$\mathcal{F}_T^*$ is described by rotation R^* and translation t^*, $\mathcal{F}_{T,i}$ by rotation R_i and translation t_i. The quality of the recovered position is measured with the residual rotation angle between R^* and R_i

$$\epsilon_\alpha = \arccos\left(\frac{\text{trace}(R_{res}) - 1}{2}\right), \quad \text{with } R_{res} = R^* R_i^T \tag{4.13}$$

and the Euclidian distance between t^* and t_i

$$\epsilon_d = \|t^* - t_i\|. \tag{4.14}$$

Additionally, the root mean square of the difference between the projected $2D$ image points $S_i^*, i = 1 \ldots n$ at the reference position and the image points $S_i, i = 1 \ldots n$ at the recovered position is given by

Two Novel Approaches to Image Guided Surgery

no.	2D/3D	# iterations	ϵ_d (mm)	ϵ_α	ϵ_{rms} (px)	joints moved
2	2D	6	9.765	0.555	10.7	vertical, angular, orbital
3	3D	4	3.798	0.396	6.6	
4	2D	4 (abort)	220.6	11.63	242	vertical, wigwag, horizontal
5	3D	11	46.997	3.257	5.0	angular, orbital
6	2D	7	16.270	0.928	16.9	wigwag, horizontal, angular,
7	3D	5	6.534	0.677	7.5	orbital
8	2D	7	6.251	0.166	6.0	vertical, wigwag, horizontal,
9	3D	6	11.635	0.796	6.6	angular, orbital
10	2D	8	27.910	2.219	11.4	wigwag, angular, orbital

Table 4.3: Overview of the conducted experiments. The table shows the reposition error in translation, in angle, and the RMS error of the markers extracted from the image as well as the used algorithm and the moved joints. Run 4 was aborted, because the algorithm suggested a C-arm movement that moved the markers to be outside the image.

$$\epsilon_{\text{rms}} = \sqrt{\frac{1}{n} \sum_{i=1}^{n} \|S_i^* - S_i\|^2}. \tag{4.15}$$

Both algorithms were tested several times with approximately the same reference position. Table 4.3 shows the details of the performed runs. The runs were aborted when the suggested movements were not reasonable to execute because they were either too small or not possible, e.g. the projected markers moved outside the image in run 4. The table also shows which joints were moved in order to get to the reference position. The camera attached to the C-arm gantry has a resolution of 1024×768, so $\epsilon_{\text{rms}} \leq 6$ is hardly recognizable when comparing the two images.

Sources for error in the system are the limited extraction accuracy of the marker points in the images and the limited precision of the joint movements. In all experiments, except run 4, the 3D algorithm converged in $4-6$ iterations, whereas the 2D algorithm required $6-8$ iterations. Similar to the convergence of the error ϵ_{rms} between the image points (cf. figure 4.26) is the convergence of the difference in the C-arm gantry orientation ϵ_α) (cf. figure 4.28), and the difference in the C-arm gantry position ϵ_d (cf. figure 4.27).

The 2D and 3D algorithm work in our test environment. The *2D* solution has the big advantage that the marker configuration in *3D* is not required. The *3D* solution on the other hand gives slightly better results, converges faster, and is more stable. Depending on the given situation the suitable algorithm can be selected. In further studies the optimal marker configuration for both algorithms has to be determined.

4.2.6 System Extension for X-ray Image Stitching

Currently, long bone fracture fixation heavily relies on intraoperative X-ray images. The limited field of view of currently used mobile C-arms is the major drawback. In long bone fracture fixation surgery, surgeons need to measure the length of the bone to be reconstructed and align the bone fragments. A single X-ray image can not visualize the

4.2 Camera Augmented Mobile C-Arm (CamC)

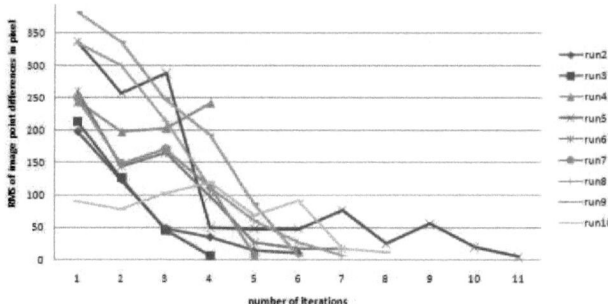

Figure 4.26: RMS pixel error ϵ_{rms} of the extracted centroids of projected points in the images.

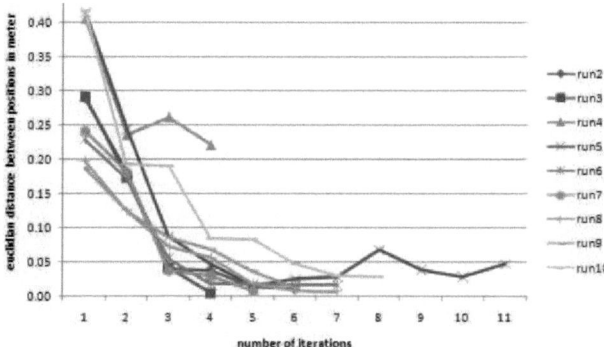

Figure 4.27: Euclidean distance ϵ_d in meter using an external tracking system as reference.

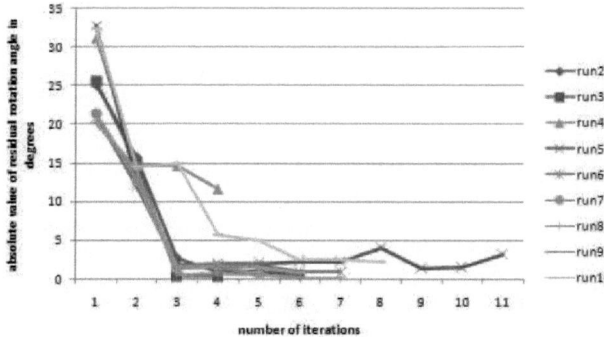

Figure 4.28: Angular error ϵ_α in degrees using an external tracking system as reference.

entire long bone, which would require surgeons to acquire several individual X-ray images and correlate them. The measurements are currently based on approximations.

Panoramic X-ray images can be obtained by stitching many X-ray images acquired by available intraoperative C-arms. A special purpose digital X-ray machine was introduced to generate panoramic X-ray images by simultaneously translating the X-ray source and the image intensifier over the patient [72]. This method requires special hardware and cannot be applied in an intraoperative scenario. For obtaining a X-ray panoramic image intraoperatively two methods were proposed using standard mobile C-arms. The first system introduces a radiolucent X-ray ruler placed along the bone of interest [264]. It uses the graduations of the ruler on the X-ray images to estimate the planar mapping transformation by a feature based alignment method and requires the user to manually select the reconstruction plane in order to compensate for parallax effects on that plane. Another method employs a radio opaque absolute reference panel with absolute coordinates placed under the bone of interest [154]. This reference panel contains a grid of radio-opaque markers and thus X-ray images can be registered based on the known geometry of this panel. However, both methods have their limitations. The first method [264] requires overlapping areas between two consecutive X-ray images to estimate the planar transformation and thus requires additional radiation, while the second method [154] is independent from overlapping X-ray regions, but requires a X-ray visible panel and does not show how to solve for the parallax effect, that is introduced if the stitching plane and the target plane are not the same. Both methods require a frontal parallel C-arm setup, i.e. the stitching plane must be parallel to the detector plane of the X-ray device.

The camera augmented mobile C-arm system can create panoramic X-ray images without overlapping X-ray images and special X-ray markers. Using the video images for stitching and finally showing their co-registered X-ray images facilitates the creation of panoramic X-ray images. The major advantage over previous proposed solutions for X-ray stitching is that it reduces radiation, does not require a frontal parallel C-arm setup, and has the capability of metric measurements. This will facilitate new applications and enable the confirmation of the trauma reduction and its quality already within the surgery room.

4.2.6.1 Method for X-ray Stitching:

Image stitching has been intensively studied in the last decades in non medical areas [232]. One central component of stitching is image alignment, called image registration, the estimation of a transformation to align two images. Intensity-based registration needs nearly identical images, which is impractical for X-ray image stitching since it will result in additional radiation exposure. On the other hand, it is hard to detect anatomical features reliably and accurately on X-ray images for feature-based registration. This is one reason why a radiolucent X-ray ruler [264] and a radio-opaque absolute reference panel [154] were introduced.

In our setup the X-ray images are registered with their corresponding video images by construction of the camera augmented mobile C-arm system. The video provides a series of images with features, in which two consecutive images are nearly identical. We first stitch the sequence of video images and then overlay the registered X-ray images onto their corresponding video images (see figure 4.29). Finally, we are able to achieve a panoramic video image, and using the associated X-ray images, we create a panoramic X-ray image.

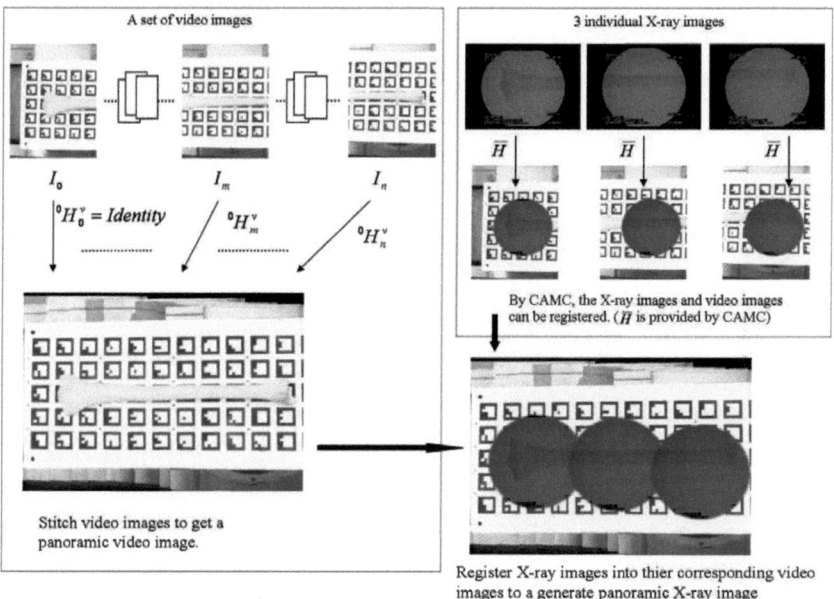

Figure 4.29: The idea of X-ray image stitching using the camera augmented mobile C-arm system and a square marker pattern. Image courtesy of Lejing Wang.

The video images are acquired sequentially. A simple pattern is used to stitch the image sequence. The first acquired image is defined as the reference (base) image, and all other images will be registered into the coordinate system of the first image (see figure 4.29). $^{i-1}H_i^v \in \mathbb{R}^{3\times 3}$ denotes the planar homography used to register each image I_i to its predecessor I_{i-1}, and can be estimated by registering two consecutive nearly identical video images. The image I_i can be registered to the image I_0 by the homography $^0H_i^v$, which will be calculated by

$$^0H_i^v = \prod_{k=1}^{i} (^{k-1}H_k^v). \qquad (4.16)$$

After stitching a video sequence, the X-ray images will be overlaid onto their corresponding video images by the homography $\bar{H}$ and thus will also be registered within the coordinate system of the first video image (see figure 4.29). This $\bar{H}$ is provided by the camera augmented mobile C-arm system (cf. section 4.2.2.3).

4.2.6.2 Parallax Effect

The planar homography that aligns two consecutive video images is represented by $^{i-1}H_i^v$. In [264] this planar homography is defined by $^{i-1}H_i^v = KRK^{-1} + \frac{1}{d}Ktn^T K^{-1}$ with $K \in \mathbb{R}^{3\times 3}$ being the intrinsic matrix of the camera, $R \in \mathbb{R}^{3\times 3}$ the rotational part, and $t \in \mathbb{R}^3$ the translational part of the camera motion. $^{i-1}H_i^v$ is valid for all image points whose corresponding space points are on the same plane, called stitching plane, defined by the normal vector $n \in \mathbb{R}^3$ and distance d to the origin in the world coordinate system. However, any structure that is not within this stitching plane in 3D space will get ghosting or blurring effects, so-called parallax. Since the $^{i-1}H_i^v$ is estimated by video images, there is always parallax effect on the bone reconstruction plane. The parallax effect will cause not only blurring, but also perturbed metric measurements.

Here, a method to compensate for parallax effects is introduced. The method relies on three assumptions: 1) images are obtained from a frontal parallel view of the stitching plane; 2) translating the C-arm parallel to the stitching plane during the image acquisition; 3) the stitching plane is parallel to the bone plane used for panoramic X-ray images and metric measurements. The first assumption defines the plane parameter $n^T = [0, 0, -1]$ and restricts the rotation of the camera to be only around the optical axis. The second one restricts the translation $t = [x, y, 0]$. Let Δd be the distance between the stitching plane and the bone plane. Based on these assumptions, especially that there is only a rotation around the optical axis, but no other rotation, we have the homography for stitching in the bone plane $^{i-1}H_i^x = KRK^{-1} + \frac{1}{d+\Delta d}Ktn^T K^{-1} = KRK^{-1} + \frac{d}{d+\Delta d}(\frac{1}{d}Ktn^T K^{-1})$. Both $^{i-1}H_i^v$ and $^{i-1}H_i^x$ are 2D affine mappings and only differ by the translation part.

$$^{i-1}H_i^v = \begin{bmatrix} a & b & x_t \\ c & d & y_t \\ 0 & 0 & 1 \end{bmatrix} \quad \text{and} \quad {}^{i-1}H_i^x = \begin{bmatrix} \tilde{a} & \tilde{b} & \tilde{x}_t \\ \tilde{c} & \tilde{d} & \tilde{y}_t \\ 0 & 0 & 1 \end{bmatrix}$$

Eventually, the missing translation part of $^{i-1}H_i^x$ can be computed by following equations:

$$\tilde{x}_t = s(x_t + au_0 + bv_0 - u_0) + u_0 - (au_0 + bv_0) \tag{4.17}$$

$$\tilde{x}_y = s(x_y + cu_0 + dv_0 - v_0) + v_0 - (cu_0 + dv_0) \tag{4.18}$$

where (u_0, v_0) is the principal point of the camera and $s = \frac{d}{d+\Delta d}$. All variables in equations (4.17) and (4.18) are known except s.

Since all images are acquired from a frontal parallel view of the stitching plane, the distance ratios and angles of the stitching plane are preserved between the images. We estimate the distance d from the stitching plane to the camera center by constructing a known geometric structure on that plane and measure its distance in the image with a known camera model. To estimate the homography $^{i-1}H_i^x$, we need to estimate Δd, the distance between the stitching plane and the bone plane. In an examplary application, the intramedullary tibial fracture reduction surgery, there are two planes: the tibia plane and the nail plane. Surgeons need to define Δd, depending on their preferences of the plane to be visualized and used to perform metric measurements.

With this depth compensation method, it is possible to estimate the homography $^{i-1}H_i^x$ directly from the known $^{i-1}H_i^v$ without explicitly computing the camera motion R

and t. This method depends on the accuracy of the estimated Δd. Table 4.5 shows the results of an experiment to evaluate the influence of perturbed Δd to metric measurement accuracy on the final panoramic X-ray images.

4.2.6.3 Frontal Parallel Setup

The frontal parallel setup (i.e. stitching plane parallel to the image plane) is the prerequisite to perform image stitching and metric measurements. However, this is not easy to establish and adds an additional challenge for surgeons to achieve an optimal initial setup. Metric rectification is performed for perspective images of the viewed plane to be able to compensate for this requirement in a non optimal initial setup. The image is rectified by a projective warping to the image that is obtained from a frontal parallel view. There are various ways to rectify images [83]. All of these methods require some metric properties or point correspondences. Since we have optical images, it is possible to construct a visible pattern with known geometry. Using this pattern all images are rectified with the same scaling. Finally, our method for intraoperative panoramic X-ray image generation relies only on the constraint that the stitching plane is parallel to the bone plane.

4.2.6.4 Implementation

A marker tracking system is able to detect markers fully automatic within the video image. In our implementation, square markers are positioned on the same plane, the stitching plane. Since these coplanar markers provide sufficient corresponding points, the Normalized Direct Linear Transformation (DLT) [83] can be used to estimate the homography $^{i-1}H_i^v$. Fixing the relative positions of square markers with known size, we are able to establish point correspondences between the points in the image plane and in their frontal positions. Based on these point correspondences, a homography is estimated to rectify images to the frontal view. We designed a pattern (see figure 4.30(a)) with multiple square markers that can be uniquely identified.

4.2.6.5 Experiments and Results

The phantom (see figure 4.2.6.5) used throughout all our experiments is constructed to have two parallel planes with an adjustable distance Δd. On the upper plane, the stitching plane, the marker pattern is attached. On the lower plane, the bone plane, we placed X-ray markers with known distances for metric measurements or a bone phantom for feasibility tests.

To determine the accuracy of metric measurements, we placed our phantom with the X-ray marker on the operating table (cf. figure 4.30(b)) such that the stitching plane deviates several degrees from the frontal parallel setup to simulate a general cases. While acquiring video and X-ray images, the operating table was moved through the C-arm and the panoramic video and X-ray images were created. We measured distances and angles between circle markers on the panoramic images and compared them with the actual values. We measured several different distances or angles with the ground truth value of 480mm or 161.0754 degree respectively, on the same image to eliminate bias error in the

Two Novel Approaches to Image Guided Surgery

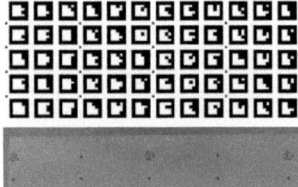 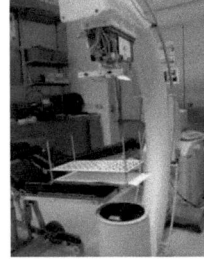 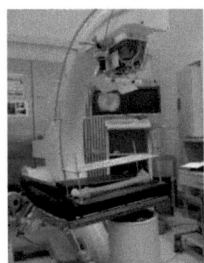

(a) The marker pattern (top) and X-ray markers (bottom).

(b) The system setup for metric measurements.

(c) The system setup for feasibility tests.

Figure 4.30: Our designed phantom for experiments. The marker pattern is attached on the upper plane. The X-ray marker and the bone are placed on the lower plane.

results. Table 4.4 shows the distance and angle measurement results. Without applying depth transformation, both the absolute and relative errors will increase as Δd increases. After applying our depth compensation method (cf. section 4.2.6.2), the absolute errors are similar to the once in the video panoramic images, and the relative errors are about constant.

	Δd(mm)	Actual value	Measured values on the video panorama		Measured values on the X-ray panorama without depth transformation			Measured values on the X-ray panorama with depth transformation		
			distance	average distance	absolute error	average distance	absolute error	relative error	average distance	absolute error	relative error
Distance (mm)	70	480	478.5752	**1.4248** ± 0.1734	476.1465	**3.8535** ± 0.0757	2.4287	477.6880	**2.3120** ± 0.1556	0.8872
	100	480	479.0940	**0.9060** ± 0.3368	473.7030	**6.2970** ± 0.1952	5.3910	478.1935	**1.8065** ± 0.1747	0.9005
	150	480	477.6040	**2.3960** ± 0.2610	466.4445	**13.5555** ± 0.0559	11.1595	476.9480	**3.0520** ± 0.0622	0.6560
		angle	average angle	absolute error	average angle	absolute error	relative error	average angle	absolute error	relative error
Angle (degree)	70	161.0754	161.2373	**0.1619** ± 0.1152	162.6729	**1.5975** ± 0.3000	1.4356	161.4325	**0.3571** ± 0.0577	0.1952
	100	161.0754	161.2895	**0.3701** ± 0.2477	163.1338	**2.0584** ± 0.0376	1.6883	161.6076	**0.5322** ± 0.3954	0.1621
	150	161.0754	161.2184	**0.1430** ± 0.1428	164.3231	**3.2477** ± 0.1879	3.1047	160.9416	**0.1338** ± 0.0515	0.0092

Table 4.4: Actual and measured distances/angles on the panoramic images in $mm/$ degrees. The absolute error (mean ± std) is between the ground truth and the extracted value. The relative error between the video stitching and the X-ray stitching.

We also evaluated the influence of perturbed Δd to the accuracy of metric measurements by applying different $\Delta d'$ to get panoramic X-ray images (cf. table 4.5). The relative error will increases with the increase of the distance between the true depth and the used depth transformation ($\Delta d' - \Delta d$). The minimal relative error is obtained for $\Delta d' = 110mm$. The reason for its deviation from the ground truth $100mm$ is that the relative error dose not only originate from the depth transformation influenced by the incorrect depth estimation of $\Delta d'$, but also from the metric rectification and the overlay of X-ray image and video image of the camera augmented mobile C-arm system. The experiment shows furthermore that an deviation of $10mm$ in the depth estimation contributes

4.2 Camera Augmented Mobile C-Arm (CamC)

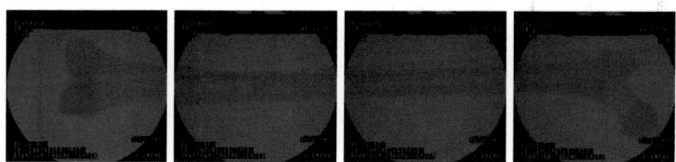

Figure 4.31: The four individual X-ray images for a single plastic bone.

to less than $1mm$ error over $480mm$ true distance in metric measurement.

$\Delta d'$ (mm) ($\Delta d = 100$mm)	0	30	70	80	90	100	110	120	130	170
Measured distance on the X-ray panorama (mean value) (mm)	473.9	475.3	477.1	477.5	478.0	478.5	478.9	479.3	479.8	481.7
Relative error (mm)	5.2	3.8	2.0	1.6	1.1	0.6	0.2	0.3	0.7	2.6
Measured distance on the video panorama (mean value) (mm)	479.1									
Actual distance (mm)	480									

Table 4.5: Measured distances on panoramic X-ray images after applying perturbed depth transformations $\Delta d'$.

In order to investigate the clinical value, we performed preclinical experiments and generated panoramic X-ray images of a bone phantom (cf. figure 4.30(c)). The panoramic X-ray image was generated from four individual X-ray images (cf. figure4.2.6.5). Figure 4.32 shows the panoramic images. Without depth transformation there are obvious discontinuous in the bone boundaries. The depth transformation compensates for this discontinuous boundaries within the bone plane.

Panorama X-ray images are a promising technology for determining the extremity length and mechanical axis of long bones online during surgeries. The presented new method is able to generate panoramic X-ray images intraoperatively by using advanced camera augmented mobile C-arm system and a planar maker pattern. Our method is independent from overlapping X-ray regions and does not require a frontal parallel C-arm setup. The experimental results show that the panoramic X-ray images generated by our method have a high visual quality and are accurate enough for metric measurements. The absolute errors were less than 1% and relative errors were even below 0.5%.

Clinical tests in the near future will show the feasibility and the advantage of metric distance and angle measurements online within the surgery room based on a standard C-arm. This will allow surgeons to ensure and validate during trauma reduction surgery the quality of their treatment.

Two Novel Approaches to Image Guided Surgery

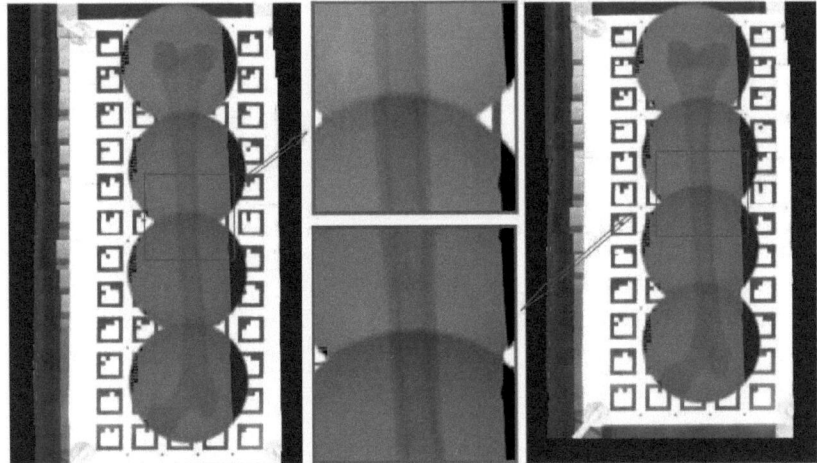

Figure 4.32: The X-ray panoramic image generated by our method. The left picture is without depth transformation and discontinuous (middle top shows) appear at the overlapping areas. The right picture shows the X-ray panoramic after applying depth transformation. This compensated for the discontinuous (middle bottom shows). Image courtesy of Lejing Wang.

CHAPTER 5

Assessment of Image Guided Surgery Systems

> For my part, I know nothing with any certainty,
> but the sight of stars makes me dream.
>
> Vincent van Gogh (1853-1890)

5.1 Conventional Assessment of the Hybrid Augmented Reality Navigation Interface

The hybrid augmented reality navigation interface described in section 4.1 was evaluated for technical accuracy including tracking accuracy, registration accuracy, data synchronization, and latency as well as for usability for navigated tasks through phantom and cadaver studies.

5.1.1 Technical Accuracy Evaluation

The accuracy of an augmented reality image overlay directly influences the accuracy of a guided task. The accuracy of this superimposition depends on tracking accuracy of the head mounted display, registration accuracy of the target points, tracking accuracy of the instruments, and synchronization of tracking data with the video data. These influences on the final user error are discussed and explained in the following subsections. Experiments are described and conducted to assess these parameters and to measure the intrinsic parameters of the used head mounted display based augmented reality system.

5.1.1.1 Single Camera Tracking Accuracy

Hoff and Vincent [92, 91] visualize the error of camera based tracking in form of ellipsoids. In their work they describe the error of the augmentation in a head mounted display within

Assessment of Image Guided Surgery Systems

a mathematical framework of error propagation. Their conclusion is that the positional error in optical tracking is always highest in the viewing direction of the camera. The orientational error lowest within the viewing direction. Thus, placing the tracking camera rigidly attached at the head mounted display within the viewing direction will ensure the highest angular precision in this direction. This results in an optimal image overlay in this direction. The head mounted display used in this thesis was a clone of the system *RAMP (Reality Augmented Medical Procedures)* originally proposed by Sauer et al. [206].

Vogt et al. [246, 247] propose an algorithm for characterization of tracking errors in marker clusters. For the head mounted display the single camera tracker relies on a well designed frame within the viewing direction. Within their studies they evaluated the usage of this single camera tracker to track tools in addition to the head mounted display. The marker configuration has to be widely distributed in space for acceptable tracking results of instrument tracking with one single head mounted camera. This results in a clinically not acceptable marker configuration. Therefore, an external optical tracking system is used. This is co-registered with the single camera tracking system by a common coordinate frame.

5.1.1.2 Registration Accuracy

Within the conducted experiments we computed the fiducial registration error and predicted the target registration error (TRE) at predefined, exemplary target points within the phantom. The fiducial registration error was estimated by

$$\epsilon_{FRE} = \frac{1}{n}\left(\sum_{i=1}^{n} \|p_{t,i} - (R \cdot p_{d,i} + t)\|_2\right), \quad (5.1)$$

where $p_{t,i} \in \mathbb{R}^3$ is the i-th registration point in the tracking coordinate system, $p_{d,i} \in \mathbb{R}^3$ its corresponding point in the image coordinate system, $R \in \mathbb{R}^{3\times 3}$ the rotation, and $t \in \mathbb{R}^3$ the translation estimated.

The fiducial registration error using our implementation with an automatic marker segmentation in the CT dataset, an optical tracking system, and a point based registration procedure [244] was estimated to be 0.28 $[mm]$ according to equation 5.1.

The target registration error was computed based on the fiducial localization error and

$$\epsilon_{TRE}^2 \approx \frac{\epsilon_{FLE}^2}{n}\left(1 + \frac{1}{3}\sum_{k=1}^{3}\frac{d_k^2}{f_k^2}\right), \quad (5.2)$$

an approximation derived from Fitzpatrick et al. [61], where ϵ_{FLE} is the fiducial localization error, n is the number of fiducial points, d_k^2 is the distance of the target from principal axis k, and f_k^2 is the root mean square distance of the fiducials from principal axis k. Both d_k^2 and f_k^2 are used for all three axes. We used principal component analysis (PCA) to estimate the principal axes of the registration point distribution.

We estimated the target registration error for all predefined points within the used phantom. The maximum target registration error between CT and tracking coordinate system was estimated to be 0.52 $[mm]$ and the mean target registration error for all defined points in the volume was 0.43 $[mm] \pm 0.03$ $[mm]$.

5.1 Conventional Assessment of the Hybrid Augmented Reality Navigation Interface

5.1.1.3 Instrument Tracking Accuracy

The tracking accuracy of the used system is to a large extent based on the camera and the marker configuration. The error of optical tracking with multiple cameras is in general a function of the distance of the markers to the cameras and the baseline, i.e. the relative position of the cameras. Recently, models for prediction and propagation of tracking errors were derived [14] and an online estimation of the error function using our laboratory system setup was implemented by Sielhorst et al. [215]. This ensures the prediction of expected application error based on the modeling and propagation of covariances. The model also incorporates the occlusion of markers and cameras (which is only acceptable using more than two cameras for tracking).

5.1.1.4 Synchronization Between Video Images and Tracking Data

The largest error in augmented reality systems is introduced by not perfectly synchronized tracking and video data [95]. In our implementation a hardware triggered synchronization signal (genlock) between video images and head mounted tracking camera is used (cf. section 4.1.2.1). Without this temporal synchronization the system will cause a perceivable jitter or swimming effect [204] that results in an errorness image overlay. The synchronization of the external optical tracking system and video cameras is based on a software framework and the clock synchronization of different PCs [220].

5.1.1.5 Latency of the System

Another intrinsic system parameter is the system latency, i.e. the duration between the data acquisition and its presentation. The lag is in general defined by the duration between the real action and its formulation. In an optical tracking system there is the image acquisition time, image preprocessing, feature extraction, triangulation, and the comparison of the detected marker with known geometric models that define the overall tracking latency, which is in general less than 50 $[ms]$. Also the acquisition of images in an augmented reality system and its processing, as well as the rendering of the medical imaging data from the estimated viewpoint require some additional milliseconds. The latency in an augmented reality system is the time between the real world action and the visualization of this in the head mounted display. This latency has a direct effect on the user performance [125, 250]. Sielhorst et al. [219] suggest a method for measuring latency using camera feedback. This method was applied to our video-based augmented reality system and did not require any extra hardware. With our head mounted display based augmented reality system, the latency was measured to be around $100[ms]$ [214]. The latency is composed of exposure time, transfer of the image data to the memory, tracking, visualization, and time to create the image on the display (cf. figure 5.1). This latency however depends on the complexity of the computations. For example complex feature based tracking methods, depth map estimation algorithms, or complex volume rendering methods will cause a higher latency.

Assessment of Image Guided Surgery Systems

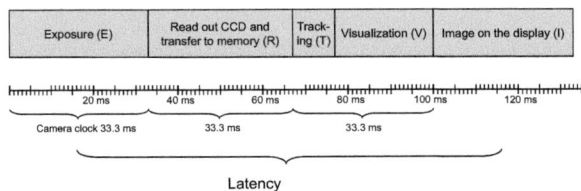

Figure 5.1: The breakdown of the latency of the head mounted display augmented reality system shows that it is composed of exposure time, transfer of image data to memory, tracking, visualization, and transfer to the display. Image courtesy of Tobias Sielhorst.

5.1.2 Preclinical Evaluation

The here used head mounted display system was used in different simulated procedures within our group [216] and within other groups [248]. Together with our medical partners from the trauma surgery department at Klinikum Innenstadt, Munich, Germany, I conducted several phantom and cadaver studies to assess the clinical feasibility of different visualization modes.

5.1.2.1 Evaluation of Depth Perception

Within our group there was a study with 20 surgeons assessing the effect of different visualization techniques on the depth perception of a surgeon. Sielhorst et al. [216] conducted this study using the different visualization modes triangle mesh, surface rendering, volume rendering, glass effect, transparent surface, and virtual window. Within their evaluation the best performance in speed and accuracy for navigation to a displayed point in 3D was achieved with the modes that have a high update rate and low latency. The most promising visualization modes were the transparent surface rendering and the modes comprising the virtual window.

5.1.2.2 Cadaver Study for Intramedullary Nail Locking

An initial cadaver study used the in-situ visualization system for training purposes for hip repositioning (cf. figure 5.2).

Motivated by the excitement of trauma surgeons to see the relevant imaging data in-situ enabled by the head mounted augmented reality system, we together designed a cadaver experiment for intramedullary nail locking of distal nails [88, 239]. For the experiment a CT scan of the cadaver was acquired. Before the acquisition of the CT scan combined Opto-CT markers were attached to enable point based registration. We ensured that the markers were attached to the anatomy such that they did not move or deform with respect to the bone structure of interest. During the study two experienced trauma surgeons used the head mounted display augmented reality system to insert interlocking screws (cf. figure 5.3(b)). Different views were presented in the head mounted display (cf. figure 5.3(a)). The favored view was not the volume rendering, but

5.1 Conventional Assessment of the Hybrid Augmented Reality Navigation Interface

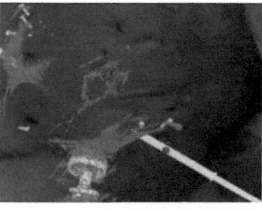
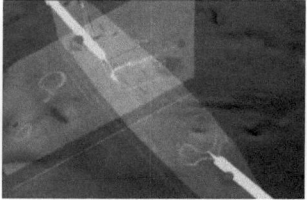
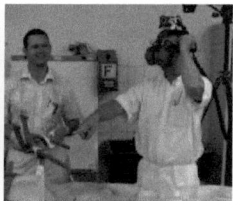

(a) Volume rendered visualization.

(b) Slice visualization.

(c) Surgeons using the system.

Figure 5.2: Volume rendered in-situ visualization and tool augmentation during a cadaver study for medical training for hip repositioning.

the semi-transparent slice view (cf. figure 5.4(c)), mainly due to the low frame rate in in our early version of the volume renderer that was around ten frames per second and caused perceivable jitter.

The evaluation of the conducted experiments showed in control X-ray images, that the interlocking screws were not positioned within the interlocking holes (cf. figure 5.4(a) and 5.4(b)). The misplacement of the screw was however not caused by misalignment of the image overlay, registration, tracking and system calibration, but by inappropriate visualization for a navigated task. In the superimposition an image overlay of reference markers which were not used for registration were permanently displayed close to the target anatomy. This was a visual perceivable reference for the target registration error and thus indicates a correct image overlay in the target region. Since these markers did not show any deviation in their image overlay, the misplacement was a clear failure of the visualization methods, proposing that a volume rendered or CT axes aligned slice rendering based image overlay is not sufficient for execution of navigated tasks.

5.1.2.3 New Visualization Concepts and the Hybrid Interface

The results of experiments using the early visualization concepts proposed new concepts based on slice navigation and its hybrid combination with in-situ visualization (cf. section 4.1.4.2). The new visualization concepts were evaluated in a simulated surgical environment. The criteria measured for a drilling task were the accuracy and execution time. Accuracy is measured as the difference between a defined target in the CT data used for the navigation and the actual position of the tip of the drill. Duration is the time measured from the visualization of the defined target point until the surgeon confirms its correct placement.

In another series of experiments, we evaluated and compared the different navigation modes within the head mounted display. We designed a phantom that mimics epidermal and osseous structures. We implanted metal spheres (4 $[mm]$ diameter) in a block of wood at a depth of approximately 30 $[mm]$. The surface of the phantom was covered with a silicone rubber compound which has properties similar to human skin and soft tissue. Combined CT and infrared retro-reflective markers were attached to the rigid part

Assessment of Image Guided Surgery Systems

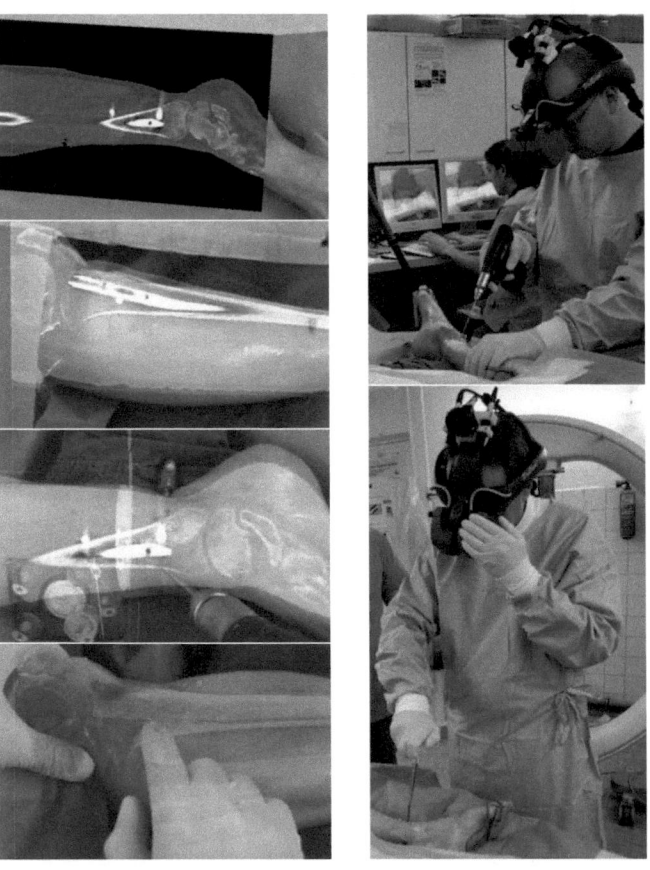

(a) Different views.   (b) Surgeons using the system.

Figure 5.3: The video see-through augmented reality system used by two different trauma surgeons during a cadaver experiment for intramedullary nail locking is shown in these images. The experiments showed that the here proposed volume rendering and CT axes aligned slice rendering is not sufficient for guiding the insertion of interlocking nails.

5.1 Conventional Assessment of the Hybrid Augmented Reality Navigation Interface

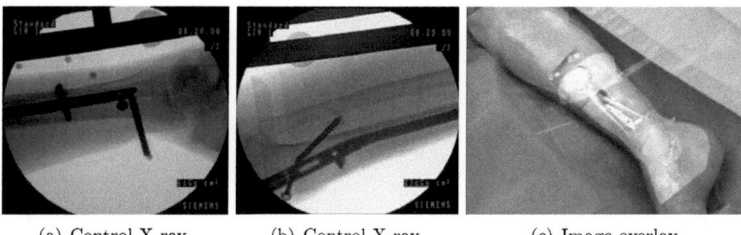

(a) Control X-ray.   (b) Control X-ray.   (c) Image overlay.

Figure 5.4: The control X-ray for intramedullary nail locking shows that the locking nail missed the locking hole. The overlay on additional markers not used for registration (red sphere) within the plane of the interlocking holes showed the validity of the image overlay system in terms of system accuracy. The misalignment of the interlocking screw was caused by inappropriate visualization.

of the surface of the phantom in order to allow fully automatic image-to-physical object registration (cf. figure 4.3(F)).

Within the video see-through head mounted display system, one of the implanted metal spheres is marked as target point and highlighted. The surgeon is then asked to navigate a tracked surgical drill to the target point using either the standard slice based navigation (cf. section 4.1.4.1), one of the three in-situ visualization modes (cf. figure 4.5) or one of the three proposed hybrid combinations (cf. figure 4.6).

The experiment was conducted by three trauma surgeons with different levels of experience. All of them marked four targets for each of the seven visualization methods, resulting in 28 measurements per subject. The mean accuracy of the three trauma surgeons for each visualization mode is summarized in table 5.1.

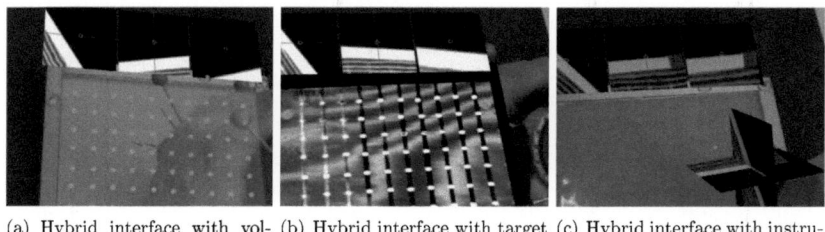

(a) Hybrid interface with volume rendering.   (b) Hybrid interface with target point aligned slice view.   (c) Hybrid interface with instrument aligned orthoslice view.

Figure 5.5: The three hybrid interfaces based on three different visualization concepts used within our experiments that evaluated their performance in a trauma surgery drilling task.

The results in terms of accuracy and speed of execution for each surgeon, as well as the distribution within the different visualization approaches lead to the assumption that the overall performance depends on the level of experience. However, a larger series of

Assessment of Image Guided Surgery Systems

Navigation	Surgeon A		Surgeon B		Surgeon C	
	error [mm]	time [s]	error [mm]	time [s]	error [mm]	time [s]
NAV	1.7 ± 1.1	128 ± 32	1.6 ± 0.7	140 ± 151	1.2 ± 0.7	35 ± 9
VOLREN	2.1 ± 1.1	134 ± 18	1.0 ± 0.4	91 ± 88	2.5 ± 1.6	24 ± 5
ASV	2.6 ± 0.8	76 ± 18	0.7 ± 0.3	50 ± 21	1.6 ± 0.9	49 ± 29
IOV	2.3 ± 0.9	98 ± 24	1.7 ± 0.6	57 ± 52	3.1 ± 2.9	47 ± 28
VOLREN + NAV	1.9 ± 1.5	106 ± 52	1.5 ± 1.3	52 ± 5	2.4 ± 0.5	26 ± 6
ASV + NAV	1.5 ± 0.2	83 ± 18	1.1 ± 0.6	50 ± 20	2.1 ± 1.5	24 ± 10
IOV + NAV	1.6 ± 0.6	95 ± 28	1.9 ± 0.5	84 ± 17	1.9 ± 0.2	26 ± 12

Table 5.1: Comparison of different navigation modes in terms of accuracy and time required to complete the drilling task. The different modes were standard slice based navigation (NAV), volume rendering (VOLREN), target point aligned slice view (ASV), instrument aligned orthoslice view (IOV), and the hybrid combinations of in-situ modes with the standard navigation.

tests with multiple surgeons on the different levels of experience have to be performed to confirm this assumption.

Surgeon A is a relatively inexperienced trauma surgeon, who does not use navigation systems in clinical routine. He performed the task with higher accuracy using the standard navigation interface in comparison to in-situ visualization modes. On the other hand he required more time with standard navigation than using in-situ visualization. Using the hybrid system, he achieved the same accuracy as with the standard navigation system but was significantly faster. This shows the advantage of a hybrid mode over a standard slice based navigation in terms of speed and over augmented reality modes in terms of accuracy. The gain in speed can be related to the intuitive usability of the in-situ component especially for inexperienced surgeons.

Surgeon B is a very experienced trauma surgeon, who uses standard navigation systems regularly in the OR. Table 5.1 shows no significant difference in the accuracy throughout all visualization modes. However, more time was needed using the standard navigation mode. This results from difficulties in finding the right entry point and drill orientation. Here the hybrid modes seem to compensate for this effect. In addition he reported after the experiment that using the hybrid modes he had the confidence of the standard navigation mode.

Surgeon C is an experienced surgeon who is familiar with standard navigation systems and augmented reality visualization. Thus, he performed the task throughout fast with no significant difference. The relatively low accuracy compared to the other candidates was due to a slightly wrong calibration of the tooltip by ≈ 1 [mm] in the direction of the drill axis. Since he was used to augmented reality he hardly used the standard slice based navigation in the hybrid mode.

In an subsequent experiment we compared standard monitor based navigation against the two modes comprising the axis aligned in-situ slice navigation and its hybrid combination (cf. figure 5.6). The same three surgeons as in the first drilling experiment with different level of experience performed the drilling task ten times for each of the three modes. The distance between the surface of the implanted metal sphere and the distal

5.1 Conventional Assessment of the Hybrid Augmented Reality Navigation Interface

end of the drill was recorded along with the time required to reach the desired target region. The time was composed of the actual drilling task and the time required to position the drill and to find the right orientation before starting the task. The results of the experiment are summarized in table 5.2.

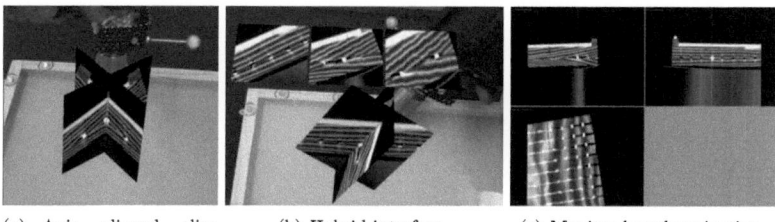

(a) Axis aligned slice view. (b) Hybrid interface. (c) Monitor based navigation.

Figure 5.6: The three visualization methods used in an evaluation to compare monitor based navigation against head mounted display based augmented reality visualization for drilling procedures.

Navigation	Surgeon A		Surgeon B		Surgeon C	
	error [mm]	time [s]	error [mm]	time [s]	error [mm]	time [s]
NAV	0.75 ± 0.68	71 ± 35	1.12 ± 0.52	66 ± 36	0.58 ± 0.44	51 ± 11
AR	0.84 ± 0.48	47 ± 17	0.69 ± 0.44	48 ± 21	0.66 ± 0.49	29 ± 8
HYBRID	0.58 ± 0.44	48 ± 14	0.97 ± 0.46	63 ± 20	0.68 ± 0.44	30 ± 9

Table 5.2: The drilling task was measured and compared between three surgeons in speed and placement accuracy. The three different modes evaluated are a) monitor based standard slice navigation (NAV), b) in-situ visualization (AR), and c) a hybrid interface of both modes visualized in the HMD (HYBRID).

The same surgeons as in the previous experiment conducted the experiments. Surgeon A required more time for the monitor based navigation than for the in-situ visualization and hybrid interface due to the more intuitive way of finding the entry point and orientation of the drill. He was more accurate with the hybrid interface compared to the in-situ visualization.

Surgeon B did not show any significant variation in speed and accuracy between all three modes. He however found the hybrid interface the most valuable for navigation since he could have the familiar information of the standard slice based navigation combined with the intuitive interface of the in-situ visualization.

Surgeon C did not show any significant difference in the accuracy performance between the three modes. However, he performed the task with all three modes faster than his two colleagues. He completed the task using augmented reality and hybrid mode in half the time he required for the monitor based navigation.

All experiments were performed within the accuracy of 1 $[mm]$ on a rigid, non deformable phantom. This is within the accuracy requirements of the surgeons for tasks like pedicle screw placement in spinal surgery and orthopedic implant positioning. Applying our methods to surgery will however have additional challenges to achieve the same accuracy for tracking and registration as in our laboratory environment.

5.2 Conventional Assessment of the Camera Augmented Mobile C-arm System

For the evaluation of the camera augmented mobile C-arm system for guided placement of instruments, we performed a series of experiments. The first set of experiments concerns the technical accuracy of the system in terms of image overlay accuracy between video and X-ray images. The second set of experiments evaluates the feasibility of the navigation aid for clinical applications in terms of accuracy for the instrument guidance, application of X-ray dose, and success in task completion. This was evaluated through phantom and cadaver experiments.

5.2.1 Technical Accuracy Evaluation

Our first experiment evaluates the calibration accuracy and thus the accuracy of the image overlay. Furthermore, it is designed to measure the influence of the orbital and angular rotation on the overlay accuracy. A pattern that is in general used for geometrical X-ray calibration and distortion measurements is attached to the image intensifier (cf. figure 5.7). This pattern contains over 300 markers that are visible in both, X-ray and video image at the same time. The centroids of the markers are extracted in both views with subpixel accuracy and used to compute the distance between corresponding point pairs. Assuming a perfectly calibrated system, no distortion or a perfect distortion correction model, and the absence of noise in the image processing, the markers will be at exactly the same position in video and X-ray images.

The makers in the video and X-ray image are detected using a template matching algorithm in Matlab. The centroids are computed using an intensity weighted algorithm. The root mean square error ϵ_{RMS} is computed in subpixel accuracy from the difference of the centroids in the video image and the transformed X-ray image between all detected points in the images:

$$\epsilon_{RMS} = \frac{1}{n}\sum_{i=1}^{n} \|p_{v,i} - H_{I_x \to I_v} p_{x,i}\|_2, \qquad (5.3)$$

where $p_{v,i}$ is the i-th point in the video image, $p_{x,i}$ its corresponding i-th point in the X-ray image, and $H_{I_x \to I_v}$ the homography that warps the X-ray image onto the video image, which is estimated during the construction and calibration of the device as described in section 4.2.2.3.

The camera positioning and calibration step was performed three times. The root mean error ϵ_{RMS} was found to be 1.59 ± 0.87 pixels with a maximum error of 5.02 pixels at one marker position. On the image plane of the calibration pattern three pixels correspond to approximately $1.0[mm]$ in metric measurements, thus the mean error is estimated to be approximately $0.5[mm]$ on the plane of the calibration pattern. See table 5.2.1 for details on the calibration accuracy.

The same experiment with the attached calibration phantom was also conducted with different angular and orbital rotations. In all angular and orbital poses, we analyzed the overlay accuracy with and without an online estimation of the homography based on four optical and X-ray visible markers. Table 5.2.1 presents the measurement errors

Assessment of Image Guided Surgery Systems

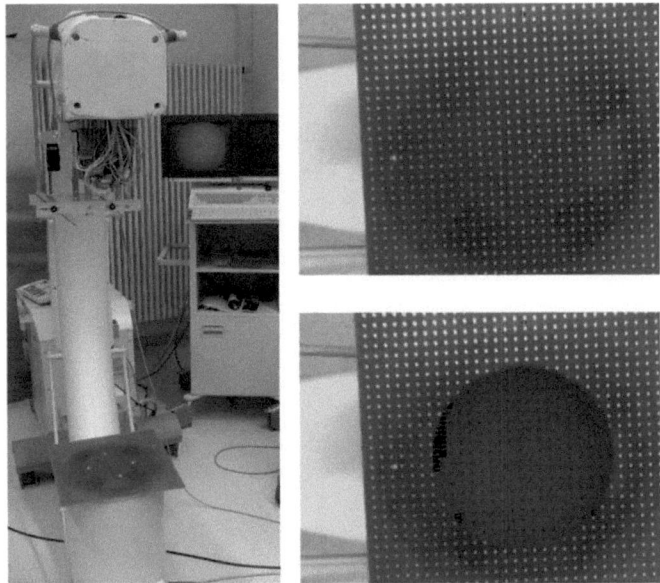

Figure 5.7: An X-ray calibration phantom is attached to the image intensifier in order to measure the image overlay accuracy. The right top shows the original image of the attached video camera and the right bottom shows the X-ray overlay onto the video camera image. In the experiment ϵ_{RMS} was estimated as the root mean square distance of the marker centroids of the pattern in the video and transformed X-ray image.

5.2 Conventional Assessment of the Camera Augmented Mobile C-arm System

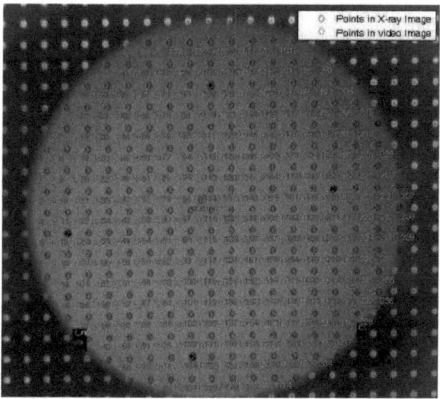

Figure 5.8: The extracted centroids of markers of the calibration pattern in the video image (red) and in the X-ray image (blue) are overlaid onto the fused X-ray and video image.

trail number	#1	#2	#3
mean	1.39 (px)	1.98 (px)	1.38 (px)
std	0.85 (px)	0.99 (px)	0.76 (px)
max	4.76 (px)	5.02 (px)	3.89 (px)
number of control points	234	237	208

Table 5.3: The difference in pixel (px) between the extracted marker centroids in the video image and transformed, overlaid X-ray image for three different calibrations.

for orbital rotations and table 5.2.1 for angular rotations, respectively. The root mean square overlay error ϵ_{RMS} was found to be approximately constant during orbital and angular rotation of the C-arm, if a re-estimation of the homography is performed at the specific C-arm position. In the cases where the homography was not re-estimated, i.e. the homography was estimated in the original position of the C-arm with no orbital and angular rotation and applied to other poses of the C-arm, the mean error of the points increases with an increasing rotation angle (cf. table 5.2.1, table 5.2.1, and figure 5.9). The experiments confirm that an online re-estimation of the homography is valid for an accurate image overlay also in the presence of distortion. Building a clinical solution one could easily ensure the correct online re-estimation of the required parameters for the planar transformation between the images. Therefore, the results of table 5.2.1 needs to be considered as a reference.

Assessment of Image Guided Surgery Systems

	0°	15°	30°	60°	90°
	orbital rotation				
mean	1.59 (px)	2.81 (px)	5.13 (px)	9.48 (px)	12.33 (px)
std	0.87 (px)	1.05 (px)	1.10 (px)	2.57 (px)	4.15 (px)
max	5.02 (px)	7.13 (px)	9.55 (px)	14.67 (px)	19.45 (px)
# points	679	239	236	232	229
	orbital rotation with re-estimated homography				
	0°	15°	30°	60°	90°
mean	1.59 (px)	2.29 (px)	2.66 (px)	2.87 (px)	2.76 (px)
std	0.87 (px)	1.07 (px)	1.25 (px)	1.17 (px)	1.16 (px)
max	5.02 (px)	5.76 (px)	6.61 (px)	6.67 (px)	6.53 (px)
# points	679	238	235	237	238

Table 5.4: The difference in pixel (px) between the extracted marker centroids in the video image and transformed, overlaid X-ray image for different orbital rotations.

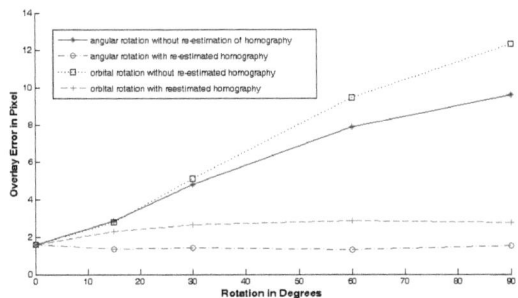

Figure 5.9: The accuracy of the overlay without the re-estimation of the homography depends on the angle of rotation in angular and orbital direction. It is independent if the homography is re-estimated.

5.2.2 Preclinical Evaluation

The system was evaluated in different phantom and cadaver studies. The first target application for the camera augmented mobile C-arm system was the interlocking of intramedullary nails. The second application domain and the focus of this thesis are spinal interventions using the system. There are conventional (open) and percutaneous pedicle screw placements as well as vertebroplasty and other needle approaches. These pedicle approaches define the primary target applications of the camera augmented mobile C-arm system and are thus the focus of the evaluation in this thesis.

5.2 Conventional Assessment of the Camera Augmented Mobile C-arm System

	0°	15°	30°	60°	90°
	angular rotation					
mean	1.59 (px)	2.86 (px)	4.81 (px)	7.89 (px)	9.61 (px)
std	0.87 (px)	0.99 (px)	0.92 (px)	1.98 (px)	3.07 (px)
max	5.02 (px)	5.83 (px)	7.35 (px)	12.54 (px)	15.21 (px)
# points	679	237	236	230	231
	angular rotation with re-estimated homography				
	0°	15°	30°	60°	90°
mean	1.59 (px)	1.35 (px)	1.42 (px)	1.33 (px)	1.56 (px)
std	0.87 (px)	0.84 (px)	0.96 (px)	0.94 (px)	1.00 (px)
max	5.02 (px)	4.41 (px)	4.95 (px)	4.67 (px)	5.08 (px)
# points	679	233	236	236	237

Table 5.5: The difference in pixel (px) between the extracted marker centroids in the video image and transformed, overlaid X-ray image for different angular rotations.

5.2.2.1 Phantom and Cadaver Studies for Interlocking of Intramedullary Nails

We performed phantom studies on artificial long bones to place interlocking screws in the intramedullary nail. The initial task is to align the C-arm in the down-the-beam position. We identified that commonly used surgical instruments need modifications in order to align the axis of the instruments under video-control insertion in the *down-the-beam* direction. The roundness of the interlocking holes in the X-ray image gives a measure how close the C-arm is to the down-the-beam position. Once, this position is reached, the camera augmented C-arm system guides the procedure by an overlay of the X-ray image onto the video image (cf. figure 5.10). The procedure does not require any additional X-ray image until the screw is inserted.

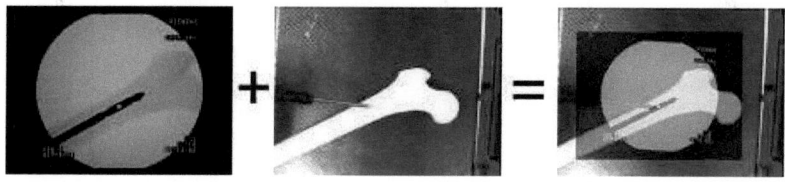

Figure 5.10: The fused video and X-ray image during an intramedullary nail locking of the camera augmented mobile C-arm system provides a guidance interface ideally using only one X-ray image. Images courtesy of Stefan Wiesner and Sandro-Michael Heining.

Following the success of the phantom studies, we performed a cadaver study for the interlocking of intramedullary nails [89]. The study showed that the surgical workflow was not compromised and the user-interface provided intuitive control of the system. The camera augmented mobile C-arm method showed a clear advantage over standard C-arm

Assessment of Image Guided Surgery Systems

based interlocking techniques (cf. figure 5.10), especially in terms of reduced radiation dose. The camera augmented mobile C-arm system enabled a robust two dimensional view to position and orient the drilling device. The drill was slightly modified to mark the extension of the drill at its proximal end. Drill-hole identification was possible in all cases.

5.2.2.2 Phantom Studies for Pedicle Approach - Vertebroplasty

For preclinical evaluation we designed a series of phantom experiments to analyze the duration and radiation time of the proposed procedure as well as the placement accuracy of the instrumentation. Therefore, we embedded five spine phantoms (T10-T12 and L1-L5) within a foam cover (cf. figure 5.11(a)). Using these phantoms we simulated the complete vertebroplasty procedure on the first lumbar vertebra (L1) as target anatomy using the camera augmented mobile C-arm system. The anatomy of the L1 within all phantoms was identical. There was no variation in the anatomy, structure, and size of the vertebra, however they were slightly differently embedded into the foam cover. The radiation dose was measured in radiation minutes and the duration to complete the task for cement filling. The task could be completed in average in $15:14[min]$ with 0.32 radiation minutes of applied dose (cf. table 5.6 for details on the experiment). The phase of cement filling however is not representative since it is not possible to perform realistic filling simulations in vertebrae without clinical indications and cavity. Thus, it was only conduced in the first series of experiments. For all subsequent eyperiments on the spine phantoms the procedure terminates after the confirmation of the correct placement of the filling needle.

The first three experiments showed a perfect placement of the vertebroplasty filling needle through the pedicle evaluated by another, independent trauma surgeon, who had no prior knowledge of the conducted experiments, using postinterventional CT data (category A according to Arand et al. [6]). Experiment four and five however showed both a very small medial perforation of the pedicle (category B according to Arand et al. [6]). Analyzing the videos recorded during the experiments confirmed that the phantom was moved between the image acquisition and the instrumentation. This resulted in an invalid overlay of X-ray and video image. As follow up of the experiments a method was implemented that is capable of simultaneously track markers in the video and X-ray image and inform the surgeon in case of patient or C-arm movement. This will ensure that any movement is automatically detected by the system and inaccurate placement of instruments caused by incorrect image overlay can be avoided. In case of motion an additional X-ray image is required to enable a valid image overlay for guided instrument insertion.

5.2.2.3 Cadaver Studies for Pedicle Approach - Screw Placement

Two cadaver studies in different levels of the lumbar and thoracic spine were performed using a percutaneous pedicle approach [87]. The placement of the screws was evaluated by a post-interventional CT and the dissection of the placed pedicle screw. The definition of the entry point was done in the X-ray image and the placement of the tool-tip and its axis alignment was carried out under video-control using the camera augmented

5.2 Conventional Assessment of the Camera Augmented Mobile C-arm System

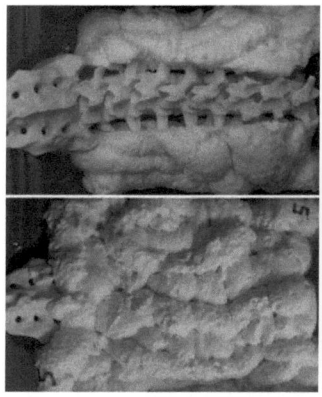
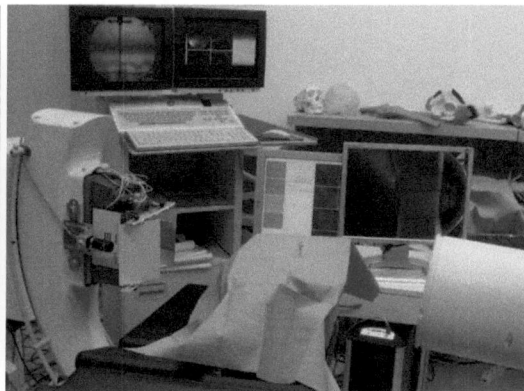

(a) Foam embedded spine phantom.   (b) System setup for the simulated vertebroplasty procedure.

Figure 5.11: Phantom experiment for the vertebroplasty procedure.

	#1	#2	#3	#4	#5
overall duration	15:00	20:10	17:00	9:15	14:46
overall radiation	0:4	0:2	0:4	0:1	0:5
placement category	A	A	A	B	B

Table 5.6: Vertebroplasty experiment performed within five foam embedded spine phantoms. Time was measured in minutes:seconds, radiation in radiation minutes, and the classification of the placement quality according to Arand et al. [6] examined by an independent surgeon.

mobile C-arm system. After the alignment of the tool axis in the *down-the beam* position, the insertion was performed (cf. figure 5.12(a)). Whenever the patient or C-arm was moved, our additionally attached X-ray and video opaque markers did not coincide in video and X-ray images any more. In this case, we acquired an additional X-ray image. Modified instruments for spine interventions were required in order to identify the instrument axis (cf. figure 5.12(b)). The experiments showed that the camera augmented mobile C-arm system provides a robust two dimensional augmented reality visualization technique for guided pedicle screw insertion. The one-time calibration was stable during both experiment series even through the mounted camera and mirror construction are not yet perfectly shielded against exposure to external force in our clinical laboratory setup. During spinal interventions through the pedicle, a considerable reduction in fluoroscopy time and thus radiation dose could be achieved. The study showed that we were close to the theoretical value of only one single X-ray image for the pedicle screw placement procedure. However, new X-ray images were acquired during the procedure for updating the intervention in terms of patient movement and implant placement control by direct imaging as well as for the control of the insertion depth through lateral X-ray images. These lateral X-ray images show the insertion depth of the instrument in the anterior-posterior direction. The amount of radiation dose was considerably less compared to the procedure only guided by a C-arm system. Pedicle identification and needle insertion was possible in all cases.

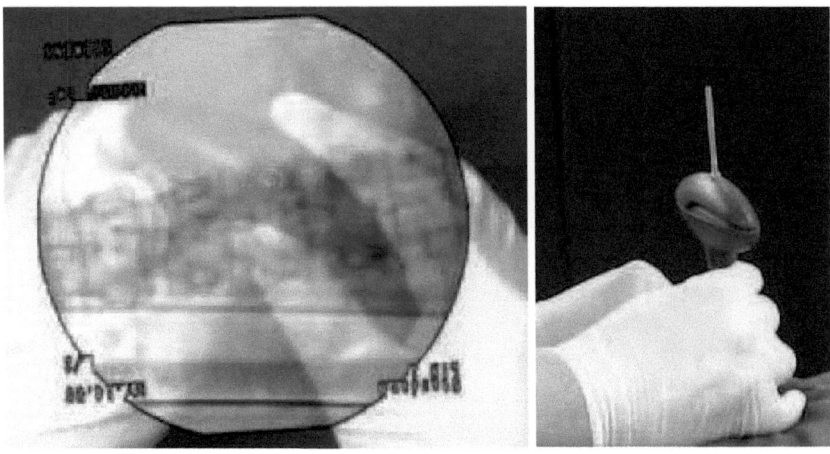

(a) *Down-the-beam* alignment.   (b) Modified needle tool.

Figure 5.12: Cadaver study for pedicle approach with a modified needle tool that is extended by a Kirschner wire to align the instrument axis in the *down-the-beam* position.

5.3 Reference Based Assessment

For the validation of medical image processing methods, a reference based approach is desired [105]. In simulations, i.e. artificially generated imaging data, it is possible to access the real image structure or transformation between two datasets (or deformation field in case of deformable registration) and thus provide a perfect ground truth for image segmentation and registration. There will be always a trade-off between the availability of a perfect ground truth and the realism of the data set/procedure. In general, in completely simulated data and procedures one has full control of all parameters of the dataset/procedure. There exist ground truth data to validate the image registration through simulations e.g. transformation, deformation field, noise, but these simulations lack of realism [106]. In real procedures it is hard to establish, control, and measure the ground truth. The establishment of a ground truth becomes increasingly complex when moving from image processing methods to image guided surgery systems.

Within image guided surgery systems it is not trivial to determine which technical system parameters are the most relevant ones. Furthermore, image guided surgery systems are extremely context sensitive. The same image guided surgery system is often not suitable for more than one clinical application domain. Concepts of existing systems have to be extended and customized for their specific needs in different application domains. Often this relation is bidirectional and it is also difficult to establish more than one suitable image guided surgery solution for the same clinical application with the optimal patient outcome and efficiency.

A method has to be established to compare the performance of systems within the same or similar environment and clinical applications. Here, the introduced camera augmented mobile C-arm system is compared to the existing standard CT fluoro guided solution for vertebroplasty procedures. The protocol has to be defined carefully in order to avoid bias in the data e.g. caused by a learning curve of the new system or surgeon specific behaviors.

Here, I propose a methodology to compare image guided surgery systems based on the workflow analysis of the current procedure, a model of the intervention, and the interpretation of models and workflow of the new and current system.

The procedure is structured in five steps as follows:

1. Perform, record, and analyze several real procedures to analyze the workflow, identify the measurement criteria, and model the surgery.

2. Design a simulated surgical procedure that is applicable for both methods, based on the model of the surgery and the measurement criteria.

3. Perform, record, and analyze both simulated methods using the same phantom or in-vivo animal study and the same set of instruments within the same environment.

4. Assess the measurement criteria and analyze the workflow of the simulated procedures in order to create comparable models of the simulated procedures.

5. Compare the methods and predict their behaviors within the clinical scenarios. In case of outliers in the data, a video documentation during the conduction of the

Assessment of Image Guided Surgery Systems

simulated procedures could enable the identification of the cause and thus justify their elimination from the data set.

In the following subsections I explain the methodology in details and apply it to the vertebroplasty procedure in order to compare the camera augmented mobile C-arm procedure against the clinically used state-of-the-art method using fluoro CT. Firstly, a clinical procedure was analyzed using a CT fluoro guided intervention. Then a generic model of the intervention was created. I created a protocol based on the analysis of the current procedure, extracted the parameters to be measured and designed a simulated surgical procedure to assess the parameters to compare the two systems. Experiments were conducted with the designed simulated procedure using both approaches. The relevant parameters were extracted and compared.

5.3.1 Workflow Analysis of the Clinical CT Fluoro Vertebroplasty Procedure

Within the CT intervention room, five vertebroplasty procedures were recorded with video cameras for analyzis with our workflow tool [2]. The clinical procedures are based on the CT image guided vertebroplasty technique as described in section 3.2.3. Two video cameras were placed in the intervention room. One camera observed the operation situs (cf. figure 3.6(a)) and the second camera showed the image data of the fluoro CT scan or spiral CT (cf. figure 3.6(b)). In addition to the video signals of the two cameras, data with two accelerometers were attached to the surgeon's wrist and recorded the motion of the arms. However, the data of these devices were not used in this work and are discussed in the Master's Thesis of Ahmadi [1].

In our workflow analysis of five vertebroplasty procedures performed by two different experienced surgeons, we had an average duration of 31:14 $[min]$ (cf. table 5.7). The recorded videos were analyzed, labeled, and synchronized using our workflow analysis tool.

vertebroplasty no.	#1	#2	#3	#4	#5	#6	#7
duration in $[min]$	32	25	22	35	37	43	24

Table 5.7: The average duration of a vertebroplasty procedure.

These procedures were recorded and analyzed to derive the measurement criteria for a comparison of simulated vertebroplasty procedures using CT fluoro guided and camera augmented mobile C-arm system. The main measurement criteria were the time required to complete specific tasks and the applied radiation dose during specific phases of the surgery. Furthermore, an average workflow of the recorded clinical procedures was used to create a high level surgical model for CT Fluoro navigated vertebroplasty procedures that remains valid throughout the different techniques e.g. using the camera augmented mobile C-arm.

5.3.2 Surgical Model of the Clinical CT Fluoro Vertebroplasty Procedure

Based on the workflow analysis, a surgical model for the vertebroplasty procedure was constructed. This was done in different hierarchical levels. Level one is a high level approach and consists only of three phases. These phases are independent of the applied technology for the procedure. The three phases are:

1. Target identification in the imaging data, i.e. the setup of the equipment, devices, the positioning of the patient on the intervention table, and the localization of the identified vertebra within the image data.

2. Tool placement, i.e. the process of inserting the instrument through the pedicle into the central vertebra cavity.

3. Cement augmentation, i.e. the filling of the cavity of the vertebra with cement.

The phases are selected such that they are valid for all vertebroplasty procedures independent of the applied technique. This means it is also valid for sole C-arm based or any other including navigated procedures. Criteria are defined to identify the start and end of each phase in order to quantify measurement criteria specific to only one phase during the procedure. To distinguish between the phases, events are defined that occur at a distinct point and mark the transition from one phase to another.

Phase 1, the target identification phase ends once the patient is on the table, all equipment that is required for the procedure is available, and the access path is identified within the imaging data. For the transition between phase 1 and phase 2, the correct placement of the patient with respect to the imaging device is considered. This is defined in both procedures by the skin incision, in the CT fluoro guided using the information of the laser beam projected on the patient, in the camera augmented mobile C-arm system by the image overlay.

Phase 2 contains the positioning and alignment of the instrumentation, as well as its insertion into the inflicted vertebra. The access path is supposed to have a central position within the pedicle without perforation. Furthermore, the filling needle requires a central position within the vertebra cavity.

For the transition between phase 2 and phase 3, the placement validation was chosen to be representative within both procedure, i.e. the final confirmation of the placement before the cement augmentation. In CT fluoro guided vertebroplasty this is defined by the spiral CT scan that shows the central positioning of the filling needle. For the camera augmented mobile C-arm system this is defined by the lateral X-ray image that confirms the correct placement of the filling needle. To define it at a distinct, uniquely identifiable point in time independent of the applied procedure, the beginning of the cement mixing was used.

Phase 3 contains the cement mixing and its application into the cavity of the vertebra. The filling process is controlled either by fluoro CT or X-ray fluoroscopy to detect any leakage during the filling process. Phase 3 ends with the removal of the filling needle. This also indicated the end of the entire procedure. Finally the band-aid is attached unguided.

Assessment of Image Guided Surgery Systems

In addition to the high level surgical model, several patterns were observed in the workflow analysis of the real vertebroplasty procedure. In phase 1 there are several loops of table positioning and fluoro CT scans until the patient is positioned perfectly in the CT gantry, i.e. the fluoro slice that images the vertebra of interest is in the focus of the scanner. Another repeating pattern within phase 2 is the instrument positioning and fluoro CT scan. The surgeon identifies the instrument on the fluoro CT scan, manipulates the instrument, and acquires another fluoro CT scan. This is a repeating pattern until the surgeon requires a 3D control through a spiral CT scan. Another repeating pattern within this phase is observed when the position can not be confirmed in the 3D spiral CT scan, the surgeon goes back to the fluoro CT mode and continues to align the instrument using the information of the needle position within the fluoro CT slices.

These three repeating patterns could be observed throughout all recorded real vertebroplasty procedures within the CT intervention room at Klinikum Innenstadt, Munich, Germany. The repeating patterns indicate potential optimization and improvements of the workflow through the introduction of computer assisted navigated procedures.

5.3.3 Design of a Simulated Surgical Procedure for Workflow Based Assessment in Vertebroplasty

For a structured preclinical evaluation a series of experiments to analyze the duration and radiation time within each phase was designed. To create a simulated surgical procedure, we embedded five spine phantoms (T10-T12 and L1-L5) within a foam cover (cf. figure 5.11(a)). For these phantoms we simulated the complete process for vertebroplasty on the first lumbar vertebra (L1) as target anatomy using the camera augmented mobile C-arm system and the twelfth thoracic vertebra (T12) target anatomy using fluoro CT navigated vertebroplasty. The anatomy of the L1 in the phantoms is only slightly different compared to the anatomy of T12, but is identical between all phantoms. There was no variation in the anatomy of the same vertebra, however they were slightly different embedded into the foam (orientation and location). Using the above defined transitions we are able to assess all phases independently and measure their duration and required radiation dose. The last phase of cement augmentation was not representative during the experiments since it is not possible to perform realistic simulation in vertebrae without clinical indications and without cavity for the filling. The cement filling is also not subject for a navigated insertion, but controlled by real time imaging and image processing methods.

5.3.4 Workflow Analysis of Simulated Vertebroplasty Procedure using Fluoro CT and the Camera Augmented Mobile C-arm System

The simulated vertebroplasty procedure was performed five times for the fluoro CT guided method in the CT scanner room and five times using the camera augmented mobile C-arm system (cf. figure 5.13). The simulated procedures were recorded with several cameras and analized to measure the criteria precisely and reproducible. The overall duration and

5.3 Reference Based Assessment

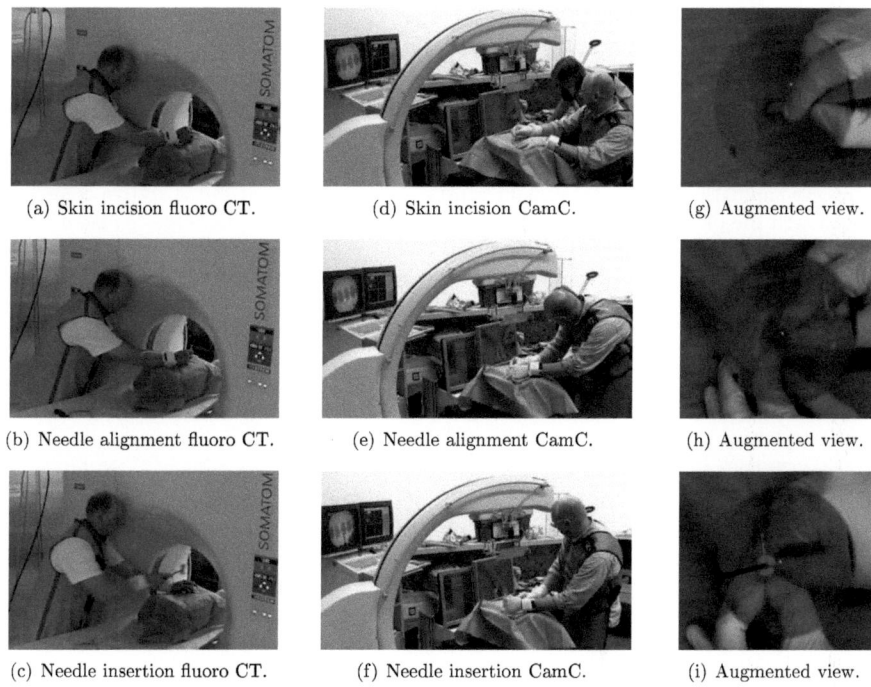

Figure 5.13: The skin incision, needle placement, and needle insertion using the fluoro CT guided procedure (left images) and the camera augmented mobile C-arm system (middle images). The image overlay of X-ray image and the real time video image facilitate instrument guidance (right images).

the individual duration of each phase was measured in seconds extracted offline from the recorded videos.

The overall duration was significantly longer using the camera augmented mobile C-arm system. The average duration was 13:14 [min] for the camera augmented mobile C-arm compared to 4:11 [min] using the CT fluoro procedure. Since the cement filling procedure was not performed within the fluoro CT procedure, this phase was excluded from the camera augmented mobile C-arm procedure resulting in 8:48 [min]. This is still significantly higher compared to the fluoro CT guided procedure. This is mainly caused by the instrument insertion phase through multiple orbital rotations of the C-arm that is needed to acquire lateral X-ray images for insertion depth control. The system setup and target identification phase is similar in both procedures. Since the fluoro CT procedure is performed frequently in clinical routine, also the learning curve has to be considered that results in a longer insertion time using newly introduced systems. The radiation showed a considerable reduction using the camera augmented mobile C-arm system compared to the fluoro CT guided procedure. Within the experiment it was hard to quantify and compare the applied radiation dose between the CT scanner and the C-arm system. Therefore, we will integrate an external dose estimation device into the evaluation process for the upcoming clinical trials.

Finally, the accuracy of the placement was measured. An observer, not involved in the surgery simulations and thus without a priori knowledge about the operative technique, evaluated the placement based on postinterventional CT scans. The clinical classification was performed according to three groups defined by Arand et al. [6]. Since the proposed scale is for pedicle screws, we slightly modified it for the classification of the canula position within the pedicle. Group A is classified by central screw positions without any perforation in any direction. Group B is classified by lateral, medial, caudal and cranial perforation smaller than the depth of thread of the screw. In our case, for canula insertion, we choose the perforation to be smaller than the needle thickness. Group C originally classify the screws with a perforation larger than the depth of thread of the screw. We used a perforation larger than the canula thickness as measurement criteria for the group C classification.

In two of the five experiments using the camera augmented mobile C-arm system there was a medial perforation of the pedicle, three pedicles were placed perfectly. The medial perforation was caused by an undetected motion of the patient anatomy that we could observe in the videos using the workflow analysis tool. An online detection of markers that are simultaneously visible in the video and the X-ray image was integrated after these experiments to detect any misalignment or motion during the procedure.

Within the fluoro CT guided procedure similar placement accuracy was observed. The experiment four showed medial perforation of the pedicle and in experiment five the surgeon required a second attempt to place the needle within an acceptable position.

	#1	#2	#3	#4	#5
overall duration	15:00	20:10	17:00	9:15	14:46
overall radiation	0.4	0.2	0.4	0.1	0.5
setup time	2:31	0:38	0:20	0:45	2:33
insertion time	8:05	14:32	13:00	5:30	5:11
filling time	4:24	5:00	3:40	3:00	7:02
setup radiation	0.3	0.0	0.0	0.0	0.1
insertion radiation	0.1	0.2	0.4	0.1	0.2
filling radiation	0.1	0.0	0.0	0.0	0.2
placement category	A	A	A	B	B

Table 5.8: Vertebroplasty experiment using the camera augmented mobile C-arm system on five foam embedded spine phantoms (L1). Time in minutes:seconds, radiation in radiation minutes, placement category according to Arand et al. [7].

	#1	#2	#3	#4	#5
overall duration	3:30	5:25	4:45	3:05	4:09
patient positioning time	0:54	1:00	0:30	0:35	0:30
insertion time	2:36	4:25	4:15	2:35	3:39
placement category	A	A	A	B	A (2nd try)

Table 5.9: Vertebroplasty experiment using the fluoro CT guided procedure. Time in minutes:seconds, radiation in radiation minutes, placement category according to Arand et al. [7].

5.3.5 Discussion of the Analysis of the Simulated Procedure

The simulated procedure is a first step towards reference based assessment of the entire procedure. On the one side, the simulation allows a comparison of the overall surgical procedure here in terms of duration and applied radiation dose. On the other side it allows to assess the phases of a surgery independently. Most preclinical evaluations only consider the assessment of the navigated phase. This however can lead to a biased result ignoring influences of the newly introduced system into other phases of the surgery (e.g. initialization and system setup). The here proposed method requires to assess the parameters independent from the used technology. In this case it was not entirely possible to compare the applied radiation dose, since no independent device measuring the radiation in the CT scanner and C-arm was used. The simulation showed however the potential of the new application in the reduction of the radiation dose, as well as its current limitations resulting in an increased duration.

CHAPTER 6

Discussion and Conclusion

> Everything should be made as simple as possible,
> but not simpler.
>
> *Albert Einstein (1879-1955)*

6.1 Discussion

In the past several image guided surgery systems found their way into the operating room. Even more projects are currently under investigation within promising research activities that have not yet found their way into a clinically applicable system.

The process of assessing the technical system parameters and the conduction of preclinical phantom and cadaver experiments is often a tedious process. A concept for rigorous assessment of new image guided surgery systems is the key for success to turn inventions into innovations. Three reasons could be identified within the scope of this thesis for the difficult transformation of research prototypes (i.e. system used in the laboratory setup in preclinical tests) to clinical prototypes (i.e. system used within the real scenario on real patients):

1. Systems are often specified without implicit knowledge of system architecture and composition, but only using explicit knowledge from experienced engineers and researchers. There is a clear lack of modeling formalisms and design patterns for building and engineering image guided surgery systems.

2. Systems are often specified by engineers, but not in close collaboration with the medical end user. This creates beautiful technical solutions, but is in general not a physician centered design. Furthermore, these solutions do in general not smoothly integrate into the clinical workflow.

Discussion and Conclusion

3. Systems are hard to assess since it is challenging to establish a reliable ground truth. Before the introduction of a system into the routine patient treatment it is almost impossible to derive its behavior in real conditions. It is an ethical question how mature a system has to be for its introduction in the operating room. This is especially critical with radical new innovations.

In the following subsections these three reasons will be discussed in details. The novel systems introduced within this thesis will be used as examples.

6.1.1 Towards the Creation of System Models

Image guided surgery systems and their components have been described in different surveys in terms of underlying technologies and application domains e.g. in [131, 183, 184, 263]. All of them identify as the major components of an image guided surgery system the images, tracking systems, and the human computer interaction. However, no model for the connectivity of the components is provided. This is to a large extent dependent on the experience of the researcher and the application engineer.

In figure 6.1 I introduce a first draft of a new notation to relate all components involved in a image guided surgery system. The central component in the proposed diagram is the medical navigation system. Each navigation system consists of a minimum of one medical information entity, a minimum of one technical information entity, and a minimum of one human computer interaction device. In general a magnitude of each of these entities is involved in a single navigation system. The relationships between these components are based on algorithms from the fields of image processing, image registration, temporal and spatial registration procedures, extraction of relevant information from the entire knowledgebase of surgical cases and patient specific data. This notation and its novel use to model and represent image guided surgery systems is proposed, motivated by the functionality of Unified Modeling Language (UML) class diagrams [201], a well known formal modeling language for the design and development of object oriented software [40, 103]. It is supposed to represent a generic approach to any navigation solutions in different clinical application domains. Instantiations of the model could visualize patterns and connectivities of the system components and algorithms.

The class diagram in unified modeling language describes different objects and components. Also their relationships in terms of role and magnitude are modeled. All components and methods of a image guided surgery system are modeled as classes and their relationship specified using different relationship patterns. In the follow paragraphs the basic entities of the model will be explained:

Class: A class is represented by a box (cf. figure 6.2). In the case of image guided surgery systems all general components and algorithms are represented as classes and the specific component and algorithms of a system by an instance of this class. A stereotype can define the category of the class or its instance. A class and its instances can contain functions and attributes.

6.1 Discussion

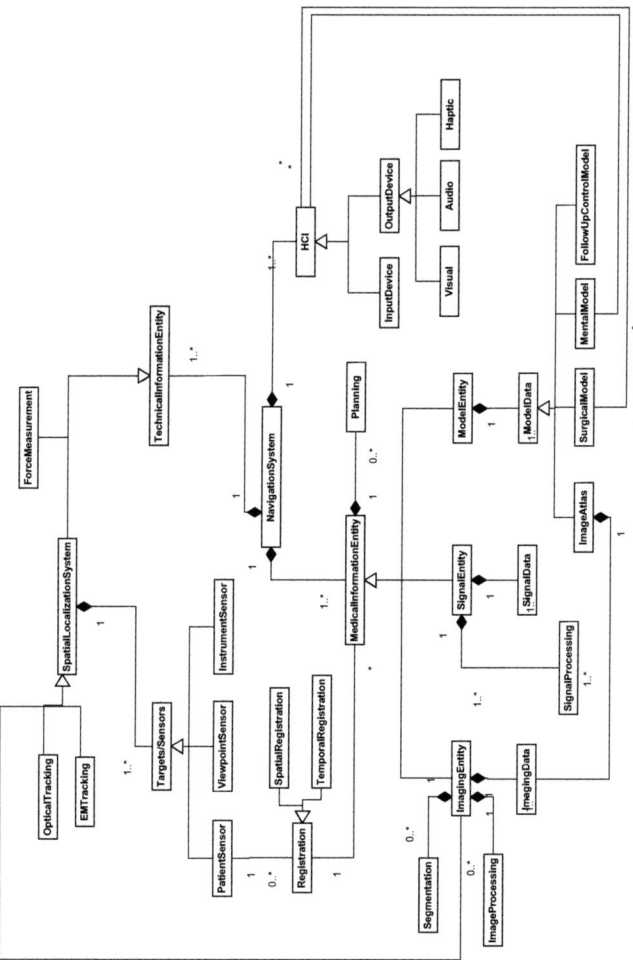

Figure 6.1: Class Diagram showing the components of an image guided surgery system and their relationship.

Composition: A composition is a relationship between two classes or their instances depicted by a black diamond (cf. figure 6.3). This means that the class with the diamond attached is composed of the other class. The numbers indicate the magnitude of their involvement. 1 indicates that exactly one instance is involved, 1...∗ indicates that a minimum of one instance of this object is involved, and 0...∗ or ∗ indicates that any

129

Discussion and Conclusion

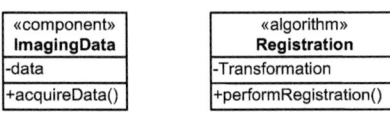

Figure 6.2: Classes for *Registration* with the stereotype algorithm and for *ImagingData* with the stereotype component. The classes have associated attributes and operations. − indicates attributes, + indicates methods associated with the class.

number of instances is optionally involved.

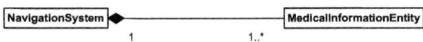

Figure 6.3: The black diamond indicates a composition. The *NavigationSystem* is composed of *MedicalInformationEntities*. The number indicates that there is a minimum of one *MedicalInformationEntity* involved and exactly one *NavigationSystem*.

Inheritance: Inheritance is a concept in the unified modeling language depicted by a triangular arrowhead (cf. figure 6.4). The parent class is indicated with the arrowhead. The child classes are refinements of the concepts of the parent class implementing specific additional attributes and operations, reimplementing or adopt existing ones.

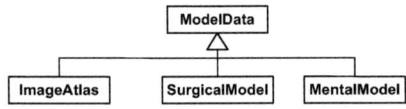

Figure 6.4: The triangular arrowhead indicates an inheritance relationship. The *ModelData* is the superclass of *ImageAtlas*, *SurgeryModel*, and *MentalModel*. A child class inherits the functionality and properties of a superclass and refines them.

Figure 6.1 uses this notation and proposes a formalism to describe a general navigation system. Every navigation system consists of a technical information entity, in most systems in form of an optical tracking system. Other instances of spatial localization system or tracking systems can be electromagnetic tracking (EMT) or medical image data, like catheters tracked in a fluoroscopic image using techniques of visual servoing. All of these localization entities have common and device specific attributes and functions. The navigation system also consists of at least one medical information entity. In general there are multiple medical information entities involved. Examples for medical information entities are preprocessed imaging data of the patient, biosignals of the patient, or models

6.1 Discussion

of anatomy and physiology, as well as models of the medical procedure and the clinical case. Finally, the navigation system consists of at least one human computer interaction concept. In a very basic version this is simply a monitor representing the medical imaging data and the spatial relationship between tools and patient anatomy. More complex scenarios implement sophisticated ways of information representation and interaction, both in advanced hardware and software. One example for advanced software concepts is the integration of the medical workflow in order to represent the required and relevant information [107, 169]. An example for advanced hardware and software concepts is the use of in-situ visualization techniques in order to present the information smoothly integrated into the current clinical procedure [238, 240].

An exemplary instance of the model is created for the camera augmented mobile C-arm system (cf. figure 6.5). The core componenets of the camera augmented mobile C-arm system are the *Image Overlay*, the *Video Image*, the *X-ray image*, the *Visualization Monitor*, and the *Control Monitor*. Attached markers visible in X-ray (*PatientSensorXray*) and video (*PatientSensorVideo*) image are used for a *Plausibility Check* and detect any patient or C-arm motion resulting in an incorrect *Image Overlay*.

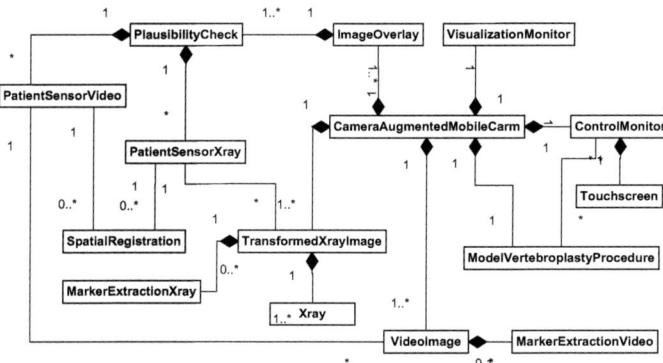

Figure 6.5: The system model of the camera augmented mobile C-arm system.

Another examplary instance of the model is created for the head mounted display based in-situ visualization system (cf. figure 6.6). The model shows the increased complexity compared to the model of the camera augmented mobile C-arm system. The *In-Situ Visualization System* is composed of two localization systems, the external optical *Tracking System* and the *Head Mounted Tracking Camera*. A *Tracking Reference Frame* establishes a common reference frame between the two localization systems. The images of two video cameras (*Video Camera Right* and *Video Camera Left*) are visualized in the head mounted display. The head mounted display provides a *Volume Rendered* or *Slice Rendered* visalization of the *Registered Medical Imaging Data*. Finally the models could be used to derive the complexity of the systems and derive design patterns for engineering suitable solutions based on approved concepts.

131

Discussion and Conclusion

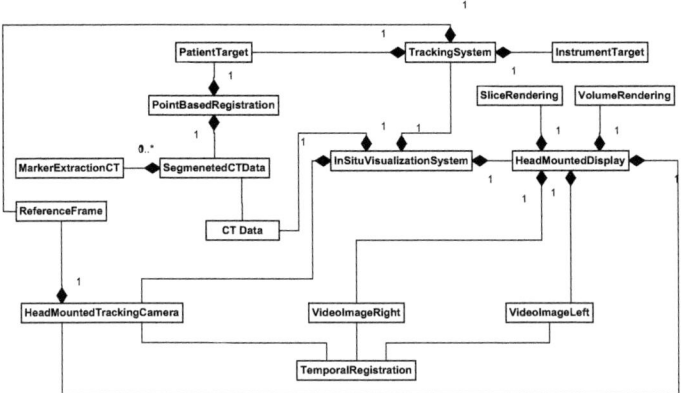

Figure 6.6: The system model of the head mounted display based in-situ visualization system.

6.1.2 Towards the Integration of Surgical Models and Online Phase Detection in the Clinical Workflow

In addition to the missing modelling methods for image guided surgery systems in the existing reviews, they do not consider incorporating models of the surgery and the clinical workflow. These tasks remain in most image guided surgery systems subject to the mental model of the physician, her/his experience, and his/her explicit knowledge about procedure specific information. Chapter 1.3 provided a short overview of the state-of-the art in medical workflow acquisition and analysis. The ideas and methods to use the acquired information of the medical workflow and surgical models for the design of image guided surgery systems and novel user interfaces is a first step towards more appropriate image guided surgery system for the optimal execution of complex surgical tasks [107, 169]. In addition, the online detection of phases in the surgical workflow e.g. [31] has further impact on the design and development of more intuitive solutions. Thus, information required at distinct phases during a surgery can be fully automatically retrieved and presented in the right form in order to complete the surgical task. This will enable context sensitive user interfaces that enhance the surgical process smoothly.

One example will be the head mounted display based augmented reality system that could propose different visualization methods depending on the phase in the workflow. Following the model of Dubois et al. [48, 49] the change in the visualization could also controlled by the distance of the surgical tool to the target location. Depending on this distance the images in the head mounted display could change from an in-situ visualization mode that gives a good overview and intuitive feedback towards a slice based navigation for fine navigation. The usage of this application specific knowledge will enable smart interfaces for surgical navigation.

6.1.3 Towards Standardized Preclinical Assessment of Image Guided Surgery Systems

Finally, the last identified reason for difficult transformation of research prototypes into clinical solutions is the lack of structured methods to assess image guided surgery systems. In section 5.3 a reference based method for preclinical assessment of image guided surgery systems was introduced. A complete preclinical evaluation of image guided surgery systems comprises the evaluation of the technical system parameters and its performance in simulated procedures within ex-vivo phantom studies and in-vivo animal studies. A first attempt was performed for the camera augmented mobile C-arm system in order to compare it to the clinical state-of-the-art vertebroplasty procedure performed under CT fluoro control. Standard assessment protocols and procedures will facilitate the creation of the required documentation for patient insurance, ethical approval, and certification. This will enable that systems can find their way easier into the operating room while ensuring the safety for patients that are within first clinical trials. There are many requirements defined for certification and conformity of image guided surgery systems. However, these requirements do not propose a methodology and a practical solution how to establish these requirements.

Discussion and Conclusion

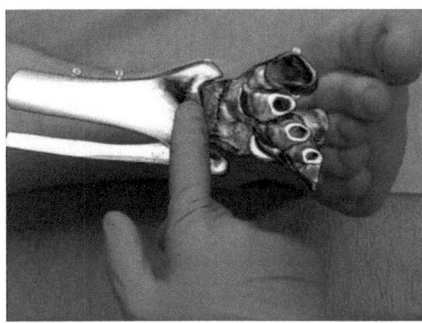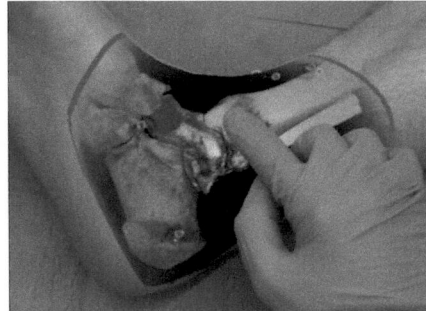

Figure 6.7: Augmentation of CT data onto my foot. Improved visualization with a raycasting technique including focus and context visualization as originally proposed by [124] and color based hand occlusion detection that runs with 30fps. Image courtesy of Oliver Kutter.

6.2 Conclusion

Within my thesis I introduced two entirely novel concepts for image guided surgery customized for applications in spinal surgery.
The first system is based on a video see-through head mounted display for in-situ visualization. Initial cadaver experiments showed a failure of standard medical augmented visualization techniques. Using the results of this preliminary experiments, as well as observations and analysis of real surgical procedures, and extensive discussions with trauma surgeons, a new concept for visualization was developed. Based on standard slice rendering concepts, a hybrid interface was developed that combines the intuitiveness of in-situ visualization with the accuracy of standard multiplanar reconstructed slice viewing. Initial tests showed that the hybrid interface is a promising alternative for visualization in image guided surgery, however the technical complexity of the system setup, including radically new devices, here the head mounted display, will slow down its introduction within the operation theatre. To completely integrate this new system into the operation room, the technology needs maturity and rigorous assessment. We are currently investigating further concepts for visualization including real time occlusion detection of real and virtual objects (cf. figure 6.7). Also the improvement of the technical setup, weight and handling of the device, as well as its smart integration into the clinical workflow have to be incorporated. Models of intervention e.g. [107] in combination with online phase detection during the intervention e.g. [31] will introduce the possibility to implicitly show the so far explicitly used knowledge and data. In general in-situ visualization based on head mounted displays proposes an intuitive and promising approach to enhance image guided interventions, however it needs maturity, reduction of system complexity for the end user, and further development towards application specific requirements derived from workflow analysis and models of surgery to find its way into the operating room.

The second system is also based on augmented reality technologies. The system extends a mobile C-arm by a video camera and provides an image overlay of X-ray and the real time video image. The overlay is realized by construction of the device without further patient registration. This system shows promising results reducing radiation exposure in everyday clinical routine for patients and surgical staff. The system was extended to meet the application specific requirements for spinal surgery. Further analysis of the surgical workflow and the creation of models of surgery could further facilitate the integration of the system into the operation room. Through their preclinical evaluation the different extensions showed that they will provide tools to augment the current clinical state-of-the-art procedures.

In order to assess and compare new image guided surgery systems, up to my knowledge, there is no standard method available. In section 5.3, I propose a novel methodology for assessment of image guided surgery system based on the currently used surgical procedure as reference. Designing simulated procedures and a detailed analysis of the workflow of the simulated surgical procedure using the standard, clinically used method and the newly proposed image guided surgery system provides a better understanding of the benefits and drawbacks of novel systems. This will support the design and conduction of structured in-vivo animal and patient studies. Furthermore, it could propose a formalism to generate documentation to support the patient insurance within clinical trials and certification regulations. The camera augmented mobile C-arm system as well as the head mounted display based augmented reality visualization system could benefit from these methodology and easier find its way into clinical applications.

The contribution of the thesis are two novel systems and a newly developed methodology to assess them. Thus, there exist two more research prototypes with promising preclinical results in order to achieve the ultimate goal to improve everyday clinical routines for better treatment of the patient. Both new systems do not yet have the maturity for their clinical introduction. However, patient trials are scheduled for the camera augmented mobile C-arm system.

APPENDIX A

Glossary

Anterior: The front of the body i.e. where the face is (cf. figure A.1(b)).

DICOM standard: Standard used for storage and communication of medical imaging data http://medical.nema.org/.

Dorsal: The back of a human body(cf. figure A.1(b)).

Iatrogenic Trauma: Trauma caused during an invasive procedure i.e. through the access path or treatment of a target region.

Lateral: The side of the body. A lateral X-ray image is refered to as an image taken from the side of the patient showing the *sagittal* plane (cf. figure A.1).

Medial: Is used to define a point in the centre of the organism or the direction towards the center (cf. figure A.1(a)).

Percutaneous: Access to the patient done via needle-puncture of the skin.

Sagittal: Is the plane that divides the body into left and right part (cf. figure A.1(b)).

Ventral: The abdominal front (belly) of a human body (cf. figure A.1(b)).

Glossary

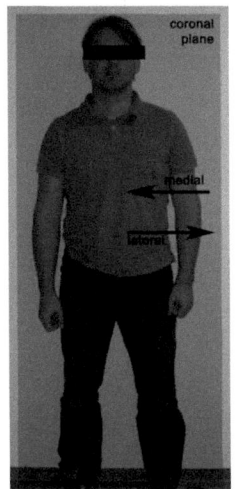

(a) Coronal view.

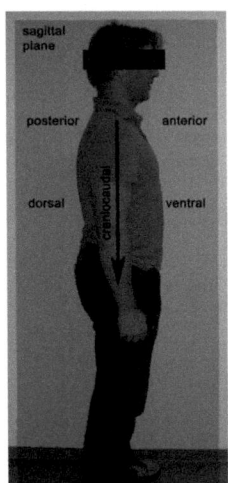

(b) Sagittal view.

Figure A.1: Anatomical terms of locations and directions.

138

APPENDIX B

Authored and Co-Authored Publications

i. N. NAVAB, S.M. HEINING, J. TRAUB, *Camera Augmented Mobile C-arm (CAMC): Calibration, Accuracy Study and Clinical Applications*, submitted to Transactions on Medical Imaging, 2008

ii. M. FEUERSTEIN, T. REICHL, J. VOGEL, J. TRAUB, N. NAVAB, *New Approaches to Online Estimation of Electromagnetic Tracking Errors for Laparoscopic Ultrasonography*, submitted to Computer Aided Surgery 2008, Special Issue of MICCAI 2007

iii. M. FEUERSTEIN, T. REICHL, J. VOGEL, J. TRAUB, N. NAVAB, *Magneto-Optic Tracking of Flexible Laparoscopic Ultrasound: Model-Based Online Detection and Correction of Magnetic Tracking Errors*, submitted to Transactions on Medical Imaging, 2008

iv. J. TRAUB, S.M. HEINING, H. HEIBEL, P. DRESSEL, E. EULER, N. NAVAB, *Two Camera Augmented Mobile C-arm - System Setup And First Experiments*, Proceedings of the Computer Assisted Orthpaedic Surgery (CAOS 2008), Hong Kong, June, 2008

v. T. WENDLER, J. TRAUB, T. LASSER, M. FEUERSTEIN, J. VOGEL, S. ZIEGLER, N. NAVAB, *Combined ultrasound and gamma probe imaging for examination of thyroid nodules*, Proceedings of Annual Meeting of Society of Nuclear Medicine (SNM 2008), Houston, USA, June 2008

vi. T. WENDLER, A. HARTL, T. LASSER, J. TRAUB, S. ZIEGLER, N. NAVAB, *3D Intra-operative nuclear imaging for SLNB in neck*, Proceedings of Annual Meeting of Society of Nuclear Medicine (SNM 2008), Houston, USA, June 2008

vii. A. HARTL, T. WENDLER, J. TRAUB, T. LASSER, S. ZIEGLER, N. NAVAB, *Confident radioactivity surface reconstruction for control of resection borders*, Proceedings

Authored and Co-Authored Publications

of Annual Meeting of Society of Nuclear Medicine (SNM 2008), Houston, USA, June 2008

viii. N. NAVAB, J. TRAUB, T. WENDLER, A. BUCK, S. ZIEGLER, *Navigated Nuclear Probes for Intra-operative functional imaging*, Proceedings of the 5th IEEE International Symposium on Biomedical Imaging: From Nano to Macro (ISBI 2008), Paris, France, May 2008

ix. J. TRAUB, T. SIELHORST, S.M. HEINING, N. NAVAB, *Advanced Display and Visualization Concepts for Image Guided Surgery*, submitted to IEEE/OSA Journal of Display Technology, 2008

x. J. TRAUB, H. HEIBEL, N. NAVAB, *Method for Calibration of a Camera Augmented C-arm*, Patent Application, EP 07024500.6 - 1526, Dec 12, 2007

xi. N. NAVAB, J. TRAUB, T. SIELHORST, M. FEUERSTEIN, AND C. BICHLMEIER, *Action and workflow driven augmented reality for computer aided medical procedures*, IEEE Computer Graphics and Applications, 2007.

xii. T. WENDLER, M. FEUERSTEIN, J. TRAUB, T. LASSER, J. VOGEL, S. ZIEGLER, AND N. NAVAB, *Real-time fusion of ultrasound and gamma probe for navigated localization of liver metastases*, in Proceedings of Medical Image Computing and Computer-Assisted Intervention (MICCAI 2007), Brisbane, Australia, October/November 2007, pp. 252–260.

xiii. T. WENDLER, A. HARTL, T. LASSER, J. TRAUB, F. DAGHIGHIAN, S. ZIEGLER, AND N. NAVAB, *Towards intra-operative 3D nuclear imaging: reconstruction of 3D radioactive distributions using tracked gamma probes*, in Proceedings of Medical Image Computing and Computer-Assisted Intervention (MICCAI 2007), Brisbane, Australia, October/November 2007, pp. 909-917.

xiv. J. TRAUB, H. HEIBEL, P. DRESSEL, S.M. HEINING, R. GRAUMANN, AND N. NAVAB, *A Multi-View Opto-Xray Imaging System: Development and First Application in Trauma Surgery*, in Proceedings of Medical Image Computing and Computer-Assisted Intervention (MICCAI 2007), Brisbane, Australia, October/November 2007, pp. 18–25.

xv. T. KLEIN, J. TRAUB, H. HAUTMANN, A. AHMADIAN, AND N. NAVAB, *Fiducial-Free Registration Procedure for Navigated Bronchoscopy*, in Proceedings of Medical Image Computing and Computer-Assisted Intervention (MICCAI 2007), Brisbane, Australia, October/November 2007, pp. 475–482.

xvi. T. WENDLER, J. TRAUB, A. HARTL, T. LASSER, M. BURIAN, A. BUCK, F. DAGHIGHIAN, M. SCHWAIGER, S. ZIEGLER, AND N. NAVAB, *Adding navigation to radio-guided surgery: new possibilities, new problems, new solutions*, in Proceedings of Russian Bavarian Conference on Biomedical Engineering (RBC Biomed 2007), Erlangen, Germany, July 2007.

xvii. T. WENDLER, A. HARTL, J. TRAUB, S. ZIEGLER, AND N. NAVAB, *Intraoperative nuclear imaging using navigated gamma-probes for tumor localization*, in Proceedings of Annual Meeting of Society of Nuclear Medicine (SNM 2007), Washington D.C., USA, June 2007.

xviii. T. WENDLER, J. TRAUB, S. ZIEGLER, N. NAVAB, *Validation of navigated beta-probe imaging with PET/CT-generated activity surfaces. New approach in radio-guided resection for FDG-positive tumors*, Proceedings of Annual Meeting of Society of Nuclear Medicine (SNM 2007), Washington D.C., USA, June 2007.

xix. P. KNESCHAUREK, J. TRAUB, *Dose Escalation with Photons - Emerging Technologies: a Physicist's Point of View*, Proceedings of the Eighth International Meeting on Progress in Radio-Oncology, Salzburg, Austria, May, 2007.

xx. R. BAUERNSCHMITT, M. FEUERSTEIN, J. TRAUB, E. SCHIRMBECK, G. KLINKER, AND R. LANGE, *Optimal port placement and enhanced guidance in robotically assisted cardiac surgery*, Surgical Endoscopy, 21 (2007), pp. 684–687.

xxi. N. NAVAB, S. ZIEGLER, J. TRAUB, T. WENDLER, *Method and device for robust inference, confidence determination of parameters, parameter and confidence visualization, and acquisition guidance based on readings of statistical processes by means of synchronized tracking*, Patent Application, EP 07010370.0, May 24, 2007

xxii. N. NAVAB, S. ZIEGLER, J. TRAUB, T. WENDLER, *Method and device for intraoperative 3D nuclear imaging, 3D visualization and image guided surgery based on pre-operative data and tracked radiation detectors*, Patent Application, EP 07010369.2 - 1240, May 24, 2007

xxiii. N. NAVAB, J. TRAUB, T. WENDLER, *Method and device for reliable intra-operative 3D nuclear imaging, 3D visualization of radioactive space distributions and image-guided surgery using radiation detectors*, Patent Application, EP 07010368.4 - 2213, May 24, 2007

xxiv. P. STEFAN, J. TRAUB, S.M. HEINING, C. RIQUARTS, T. SIELHORST, E. EULER, AND N. NAVAB, *Hybrid navigation interface: a comparative study*, in Proceedings of Bildverarbeitung fuer die Medizin (BVM 2007), Munich, Germany, March 2007, pp. 81–86.

xxv. J. TRAUB, S. KAUR, P. KNESCHAUREK, AND N. NAVAB, *Evaluation of Electromagnetic Error Correction Methods*, in Proceedings of Bildverarbeitung fuer die Medizin (BVM 2007), Munich, Germany, March 2007, pp. 363–367.

xxvi. T. KLEIN, S. BENHIMANE, J. TRAUB, S.M. HEINING, E. EULER, AND N. NAVAB, *Interactive Guidance System for C-arm Repositioning without Radiation*, in Proceedings of Bildverarbeitung fuer die Medizin (BVM 2007), Munich, Germany, March 2007, pp. 21–25.

Authored and Co-Authored Publications

xxvii. O. KISHENKOV, T. WENDLER, J. TRAUB, S. ZIEGLER, AND N. NAVAB, *Method for projecting functional 3D information onto anatomic surfaces: Accuracy improvement for navigated 3D beta-probes*, in Proceedings of Bildverarbeitung fuer die Medizin (BVM 2007), Munich, Germany, March 2007, pp. 66–70.

xxviii. N. NAVAB, S. ZIEGLER, J. TRAUB, T. WENDLER, *Paid, claims amended Method and device for 3D acquisition, 3D visualization and computer guided surgery using nuclear probes*, Patent Application, PCT/EP 2007/001678, Feb. 27, 2007

xxix. J. TRAUB, J. MUCH, A. SCHNEIDER, F. PELTZ, H. HAUTMANN, AND N. NAVAB, *User interface for electromagnetic navigated bronchoscopy*, 5. Jahrestagung der Deutschen Gesellschaft für Computer-und Roboter-Assistierte Chirurgie (CURAC 2006), Hannover, Germany, September 2006.

xxx. T. WENDLER, J. TRAUB, S. ZIEGLER, AND N. NAVAB, *Navigated three dimensional beta probe for optimal cancer resection*, Proceedings of Medical Image Computing and Computer-Assisted Intervention (MICCAI 2006), Copenhagen, Denmark, October 2006, pp. 561–569.

xxxi. J. TRAUB, P. STEFAN, S.M. HEINING, T. SIELHORST, C. RIQUARTS, E. EULER, AND N. NAVAB, *Hybrid navigation interface for orthopedic and trauma surgery*, in Proceedings of Medical Image Computing and Computer-Assisted Intervention (MICCAI 2006), Copenhagen, Denmark, October 2006, pp. 373–380.

xxxii. J. TRAUB, P. STEFAN, S.M. HEINING, T. SIELHORST, C. RIQUARTS, E. EULER, AND N. NAVAB, *Towards a Hybrid Navigation Interface: Comparison of a Slice Based Navigation System with In-situ Visualization*, in Proceedings of International Workshop on Medical Imaging and Augmented Reality (MIAR 2006), Shanghai, China, August, 2006, pp. 179–186.

xxxiii. S.M. HEINING, P. STEFAN, L. OMARY, S. WIESNER, T. SIELHORST, N. NAVAB, F. SAUER, E. EULER, W. MUTSCHLER, AND J. TRAUB, *Evaluation of an in-situ visualization system for navigated trauma surgery*, in Journal of Biomechanics, Vol. 39, Suppl. 1, 2006, pp. 209.

xxxiv. J. TRAUB, P. STEFAN, S.M. HEINING, T. SIELHORST, C. RIQUARTS, E. EULER, AND N. NAVAB, *Stereoscopic augmented reality navigation for trauma surgery: cadaver experiment and usability study*, International Journal of Computer Assisted Radiology and Surgery, Vol. 1, Suppl. 1, 2006, pp. 30–31.

xxxv. T. SIELHORST, M. FEUERSTEIN, J. TRAUB, O. KUTTER, AND N. NAVAB, *CAMPAR: A software framework guaranteeing quality for medical augmented reality*, International Journal of Computer Assisted Radiology and Surgery, Vol. 1, Suppl. 1, 2006, pp. 29–30.

xxxvi. S.M. HEINING, P. STEFAN, F. SAUER, E. EULER, N. NAVAB, AND J. TRAUB, *Evaluation of an in-situ visualization system for navigated trauma surgery*, in Proceedings of The 6th Computer Assisted Orthopaedic Surgery (CAOS 2006), Montreal, Canada, June, 2006.

xxxvii. J. TRAUB, S. WIESNER, M. FEUERSTEIN, H. FEUSSNER, AND N. NAVAB, *Evaluation of calibration methods for laparoscope augmentation*, in 4. Jahrestagung der Deutschen Gesellschaft für Computer-und Roboter-Assistierte Chirurgie (CURAC 2005), Berlin, Germany, September 2005.

xxxviii. B. OLBRICH, J. TRAUB, S. WIESNER, A. WIECHERT, H. FEUSSNER, AND N. NAVAB, *Respiratory Motion Analysis: Towards Gated Augmentation of the Liver*, in Proceedings of Computer Assisted Radiology and Surgery (CARS 2005), Berlin, Germany, June 2005, pp. 248–253.

xxxix. R. BAUERNSCHMITT, M. FEUERSTEIN, E. SCHIRMBECK, J. TRAUB, G. KLINKER, S. WILDHIRT, AND R. LANGE, *Improved preoperative planning in robotic heart surgery*, in IEEE Proceedings of Computers in Cardiology (CinC 2004), Chicago, USA, Septemper 2004, pp. 773–776.

xl. J. TRAUB, M. FEUERSTEIN, M. BAUER, E. U. SCHIRMBECK, H. NAJAFI, R. BAUERNSCHMITT, AND G. KLINKER, *Augmented reality for port placement and navigation in robotically assisted minimally invasive cardiovascular surgery*, in Computer Assisted Radiology and Surgery (CARS 2004), Chicago, USA, June 2004, pp. 735–740.

xli. T. SIELHORST, J. TRAUB, AND N. NAVAB, *The AR Apprenticeship: Replication and Omnidirectional Viewing of Subtle Movements*, in Proceedings of IEEE and ACM International Symposium on Mixed and Augmented Reality (ISMAR 2004), Arlington, VA, USA, 2004, pp. 290–291.

References

[1] S.-A. AHMADI, *Discovery and detection of surgical activity in percutaneous vertebroplasty*, master's thesis, Technische Universität München, 2008.

[2] S.-A. AHMADI, T. SIELHORST, R. STAUDER, M. HORN, H. FEUSSNER, AND N. NAVAB, *Recovery of surgical workflow without explicit models*, in Proc. Int'l Conf. Medical Image Computing and Computer Assisted Intervention (MICCAI), 2006, pp. 420–428.

[3] L. AMIOT, K. LANG, M. PUTZIER, H. ZIPPEL, AND H. LABELLE, *Comparative results between conventional and computer-assisted pedicle screw installation in the thoracic, lumbar, and sacral spine*, Spine, 25 (2000), pp. 606–614.

[4] L.-P. AMIOT AND F. POULIN, *Computed tomography-based navigation for hip, knee, and spine surgery*, Clinical Orthopaedics & Related Research, 421 (2004), pp. 77–86.

[5] H. ANGER, *A new instrument for mapping gamma-ray emitters*, in Biology and Medicine Quarterly Report UCRL, no. 38, 1957.

[6] M. ARAND, E. HARTWIG, D. HEBOLD, L. KINZL, AND F. GEBHARD, *Präzisionsanalyse navigationsgestützt implantierter thorakaler und lumbaler pedikelschrauben*, Unfallchirurg, 104 (2001), pp. 1076–1081.

[7] M. ARAND, M. SCHEMPF, D. HEBOLD, S. TELLER, L. KINZL, AND F. GEBHARD, *Präzision der navigationsgestützten chirurgie an der brust- und lendenwirbelsäule*, Unfallchirurg, 106 (2003), pp. 899–906.

[8] K. S. ARUN, T. S. HUANG, AND S. D. BLOSTEIN, *Least-squares fitting of two 3-d point sets*, IEEE Trans. Pattern Anal. Machine Intell., 9 (1987), pp. 698–700.

[9] T. AUER AND A. PINZ, *The integration of optical and magnetic tracking for multi-user augmented reality*, Computer & Graphics, 23 (1999), pp. 805–808.

References

[10] R. T. AZUMA, *A survey of augmented reality*, Presence: Teleoperators and Virtual Environments, 6 (1997), pp. 355–385.

[11] R. T. AZUMA, Y. BAILLOT, R. BEHRINGER, S. FEINER, S. JULIER, AND B. MACINTYRE, *Recent advances in augmented reality*, IEEE Computer Graphics and Applications, 21 (2001), pp. 34–47.

[12] M. BAJURA, H. FUCHS, AND R. OHBUCHI, *Merging virtual objects with the real world: seeing ultrasound imagery within the patient*, in Proceedings of the 19th annual conference on Computer graphics and interactive techniques, ACM Press, 1992, pp. 203–210.

[13] M. BAUER, M. SCHLEGEL, D. PUSTKA, N. NAVAB, AND G. KLINKER, *Predicting and estimating the accuracy of vision-based optical tracking systems*, in Proc. IEEE and ACM Int'l Symp. on Mixed and Augmented Reality (ISMAR), Santa Barbara (CA), USA, October 2006, pp. 43–51.

[14] M. A. BAUER, *Tracking Errors in Augmented Reality*, PhD thesis, Technische Universität München, 2007.

[15] M. BAUMHAUER, M. FEUERSTEIN, H.-P. MEINZER, AND J. RASSWEILER, *Navigation in endoscopic soft tissue surgery: Perspectives and limitations*, Journal of Endourology, 22 (2008), pp. 1–16.

[16] R. BEISSE, M. POTULSKI, AND V. BÜHREN, *Thoracoscopic assisted anterior fusion in fractures of the thoracic and lumbar spine*, Orthop. Traumatol., 7 (1999), pp. 54–66.

[17] R. BEISSE, M. POTULSKI, AND V. BÜHREN, *Endoscopic techniques for the management of spinal trauma*, European Journal of Trauma, 25 (2001), pp. 275–291.

[18] J. M. BENLLOCH, M. ALCANIZ, B. ESCAT, M. M. FERNANDEZ, M. GIMENEZ, R. GOMEZ, V. GRAU, C. LERCHE, J. L. PALMERO, N. PAVON, M. RAFECAS, F. SANCHEZ, AND D. VERA, *The gamma functional navigator*, IEEE Trans Nucl Sci, 51 (2004), pp. 682–689.

[19] G. BERCI AND K. A. FORDE, *History of endoscopy - what lessons have we learned from the past?*, Surgical Endoscopy, 14 (2002), pp. 5–15.

[20] P. J. BESL AND N. D. MCKAY, *A method for registration of 3-d shapes*, IEEE Trans. Pattern Anal. Machine Intell., 14 (1992), pp. 239–256.

[21] C. BICHLMEIER AND N. NAVAB, *Virtual window for improved depth perception in medical ar*, in AMIARCS - Virtual Window for Improved Depth Perception in Medical AR, Copenhagen, Denmark, Oct. 2006, MICCAI Society.

[22] C. BICHLMEIER, M. RUSTAEE, AND S. H. NAD N. NAVAB, *Virtually extended surgical drilling device: Virtual mirror for navigated spine surgery*, in Proc. Int'l

Conf. Medical Image Computing and Computer Assisted Intervention (MICCAI), 2007.

[23] C. BICHLMEIER, F. WIMMER, H. SANDRO MICHAEL, AND N. NASSIR, *Contextual anatomic mimesis: Hybrid in-situ visualization method for improving multi-sensory depth perception in medical augmented reality*, in Proc. IEEE and ACM Int'l Symp. on Mixed and Augmented Reality (ISMAR), Nov. 2007, pp. 129–138.

[24] W. BIRKFELLNER, *Tracking Systems in Surgical Navigation*, PhD thesis, Department of Biomedical Engineering and Physics, General Hospital, University of Vienna, 2000.

[25] W. BIRKFELLNER, M. FIGL, K. HUBER, F. WATZINGER, F. WANSCHITZ, J. HUMMEL, R. HANEL, W. GREIMEL, P. HOMOLKA, R. EWERS, AND H. BERGMANN, *A head-mounted operating binocular for augmented reality visualization in medicine - design and initial evaluation*, IEEE Trans. Med. Imag., 21 (2002), pp. 991–997.

[26] W. BIRKFELLNER, F. WATZINGER, F. WANSCHITZ, G. ENISLIDIS, M. TRUPPE, R. EWERS, AND H. BERGMANN, *Concepts and results in the development of a hybrid tracking system for cas*, in Proceedings of the First International Conference of Medical Image Computing and Computer-Assisted Intervention (MICCAI), I. W. M. Wells, A. C. F. Colchester, and S. L. Delp, eds., vol. 1496 of Lecture Notes in Computer Science, Cambridge, MA, USA, October 1998, pp. 343–351.

[27] W. BIRKFELLNER, F. WATZINGER, F. WANSCHITZ, R. EWERS, AND H. BERGMANN, *Calibration of tracking systems in a surgical environment*, IEEE Trans. Med. Imag., 17 (1998).

[28] G. BISHOP, G. WELCH, AND B. D. ALLEN, *Course 11 – tracking: Beyond 15 minutes of thought*. SIGGRAPH, 2001.

[29] P. BLACK, T. MORIARTY, A. EBEN, P. STIEG, E. WOODARD, P. L. GLEASON, C. MARTIN, R. KIKINIS, R. SCHWARTZ, AND F. JOLESZ, *Development and implementation of intraoperative magnetic resonance imaging and its neurosurgical applications*, Neurosurgery Online, 41 (1997), pp. 831–845.

[30] M. BLACKWELL, F. MORGAN, AND I. A.M. DI GIOIA, *Augmented reality and its future in orthopaedics*, Clinical Orthopaedics and Related Research, (1998).

[31] T. BLUM, N. PADOY, H. FEUSSNER, AND N. NAVAB, *Workflow mining for visualization and analysis of surgeries*, Proceedings of Computer Assisted Radiology and Surgery (CARS 2008), 22nd International Congress and Exhibition, Barcelona, Spain, June 2008 (to appear), (2008).

[32] S. A. BOPPART, T. F. DEUTSCH, AND D. W. RATTNER, *Optical imaging technology in minimally invasive surgery – current status and future directions*, Surgical Endoscopy, 13 (1999), pp. 718–722.

References

[33] B. M. BOSZCZYK, M. BIERSCHNEIDER, S. PANZER, W. PANZER, R. HARSTALL, K. SCHMID, AND H. JAKSCHE, *Fluoroscopic radiation exposure of the kyphoplasty patient*, European Spine Journal, 15 (2006), pp. 347 – 355.

[34] Y. BOYKOV, O. VEKSLER, AND R. ZABIH, *Fast approximate energy minimization via graph cuts*, IEEE transactions on Pattern Analysis and Machine Intelligence (PAMI), 23 (2001), pp. 1222–1239.

[35] D. J. BRENNER AND E. J. HALL, *Computed tomography - an increasing source of radiation exposure*, The New England Journal of Medicine, 357 (2007), pp. 2277–2284.

[36] S. BRITZ-CUNNINGHAM AND S. ADELSTEIN, *Molecular targeting with radionuclides: state of the science*, Journal of Nuclear Medicine, 44 (2003), pp. 1945–1961.

[37] D. W. BRODWATER, BRIAN K.AND ROBERTS, T. NAKAJIMA, E. M. FRIETS, AND J. W. STROHBEHN, *Extracranial application of the frameless stereotactic operating microscope: Experience with lumbar spine*, Neurosurgery, 32 (1993), pp. 209–213.

[38] F. P. BROOKS, *The Mythical Man-Month: Essays on Software Engineering*, Addison-Wesley Professional, 2 edition ed., 1995.

[39] A. M. BRUCKSTEIN, R. J. HOLT, T. S. HUANG, AND A. N. NETRAVALI, *"optimum fiducials under weak perspective projection*, in 7th IEEE International Conference on Computer Vision ICCV'99, Kerkyra, Greece, Sept. 1999, pp. 67–72.

[40] B. BRUEGGE AND A. H. DUTOIT, *Object-Oriented Software Engineering: Using UML, Patterns and Java, Second Edition*, Prentice-Hall, Inc., Upper Saddle River, NJ, USA, 2003.

[41] O. BURGERT, T. NEUMUTH, F. LEMPP, R. MUDUNURI, J. MEIXENSBERGER, G. STRAUSS, A. DIETZ, P. JANNIN, AND H. U. LEMKE, *Linking top-level ontologies and surgical workflows*, International Journal of Computer Assisted Radiology and Surgery, 1 (2006), pp. 437–438.

[42] F. CHASSAT AND S. LAVALLEE, *Experimental protocol of accuracy evaluation of 6-d localizers for computer-integrated surgery: Application to four optical localizers*, in Proceedings of the First International Conference of Medical Image Computing and Computer-Assisted Intervention (MICCAI), I. W. M. Wells, A. C. F. Colchester, and S. L. Delp, eds., vol. 1496 of Lecture Notes in Computer Science, Cambridge, MA, USA, October 1998, Springer, pp. 277–285.

[43] K. CHINZEI, N. HATA, F. JOLESZ, AND R. KIKINIS, *MR Compatible Surgical Assist Robot: System Integration and Preliminary Feasibility Study*, in Medical Image Computing and Computer Assisted Intervention (MICCAI), vol. 1935, Springer, 2000, pp. 921–933.

[44] K. CLEARY AND A. KINSELLA, *Or2020: the operating room of the future*, Journal of laparoendoscopic & advanced surgical techniques. Part A, 15 (2005), pp. 497–573.

[45] H. J. W. DAM, *The new marvel in photography*, McClure's Magazine, 6 (1896), pp. 403–414.

[46] A. M. DIGIOIA, B. JARAMAZ, F. PICARD, AND L.-P. NOLTE, eds., *Computer and Robotic Assisted Hip and Knee Surgery*, Oxford University Press, 2004.

[47] M. DOETTER, *Fluoroskopiebasierte Navigation zur intraoperativen Unterstützung orthopädischer Eingriffe*, PhD thesis, Technischen Universität München, 2005.

[48] E. DUBOIS, L. NIGAY, J. TROCCAZ, L. CARRAT, AND O. CHAVANON, *A methodological tool for computer-assisted surgery interface design: its application to computer-assisted pericardial puncture*, in In Proceedings of Medicine Meets Virtual Reality, 2001.

[49] E. DUBOIS, L. NIGAY, J. TROCCAZ, O. CHAVANON, AND L. CARRAT, *Classification space for augmented surgery, an augmented reality case study*, in in Proceedings of Interact, 1999, pp. 353–359.

[50] P. J. EDWARDS, L. G. JOHNSON, D. J. HAWKES, M. R. FENLON, A. J. STRONG, AND M. J. GLEESON, *Clinical experience and perception in stereo augmented reality surgical navigation*, in Proceesings of Medical Imaging and Augmented Reality: Second International Workshop, MIAR 2004, Beijing, China, August 19-20, 2004., 2004, pp. 369–376.

[51] H. ELHAWARY, A. ZIVANOVIC, B. DAVIES, AND M. LAMPÉRTH, *A Review of Magnetic Resonance Imaging Compatible Manipulators in Surgery*, Proceedings of the Institution of Mechanical Engineers, Part H: Journal of Engineering in Medicine, 220 (2006), pp. 413–424.

[52] E. EULER, S. HEINING, C. RIQUARTS, AND W. MUTSCHLER, *C-arm-based three-dimensional navigation: a preliminary feasibility study*, Computer Aided Surgery, 8 (2003), pp. 35–41.

[53] O. FAUGERAS, *Three-Dimensional Computer Vision. A Geometric Viewpoint*, Artificial Intelligence, MIT Press, 2001.

[54] L. FELDKAMP, L. DAVIES, AND J. KRESS, *Practical cone-beam proof algorithm*, J. Opt. Soc. Am., 6 (1984), pp. 612–619.

[55] M. FEUERSTEIN, T. MUSSACK, S. M. HEINING, AND N. NAVAB, *Intraoperative laparoscope augmentation for port placement and resection planning in minimally invasive liver resection*, IEEE Trans. Med. Imag., 27 (2008), pp. 355–369.

[56] M. FEUERSTEIN, T. REICHL, J. VOGEL, A. SCHNEIDER, H. FEUSSNER, AND N. NAVAB, *Magneto-optic tracking of a flexible laparoscopic ultrasound transducer*

References

for laparoscope augmentation, in Proc. Int'l Conf. Medical Image Computing and Computer Assisted Intervention (MICCAI), N. Ayache, S. Ourselin, and A. Maeder, eds., vol. 4791 of Lecture Notes in Computer Science, Brisbane, Australia, October/November 2007, Springer-Verlag, pp. 458–466.

[57] M. FEUERSTEIN, T. REICHL, J. VOGEL, J. TRAUB, AND N. NAVAB, *Magneto-optic tracking of flexible laparoscopic ultrasound: Model-based online detection and correction of magnetic tracking errors*, (submitted to) IEEE Transactions on Medical Imaging, (2008).

[58] ———, *New approaches to online estimation of electromagnetic tracking errors for laparoscopic ultrasonography*, (to appear in) Computer Assisted Surgery, MICCAI 07 Special Issue (2008).

[59] M. FIGL, C. EDE, J. HUMMEL, F. WANSCHITZ, R. EWERS, H. BERGMANN, AND W. BIRKFELLNER, *A fully automated calibration method for an optical see-through head-mounted operating microscope with variable zoom and focus*, IEEE Trans. Med. Imag., 24 (2005), pp. 1492–1499.

[60] G. S. FISCHER, A. DEGUET, D. SCHLATTMAN, R. TAYLOR, L. FAYAD, S. J. ZINREICH, AND G. FICHTINGER, *Mri image overlay: Applications to arthrography needle insertion*, in Medicine Meets Virtual Reality (MMVR) 14, 2006.

[61] J. M. FITZPATRICK, J. B. WEST, AND C. R. MAURER, JR., *Predicting error in rigid-body point-based registration*, IEEE Trans. Med. Imag., 14 (1998), pp. 694–702.

[62] K. FOLEY, D. SIMON, AND Y. RAMPERSAUD, *Virtual fluoroscopy*, Operative Techniques in Orthopaedics, 10 (2000), pp. 77–81.

[63] K. FOLEY, D. SIMON, AND Y. RAMPERSAUD, *Virtual fluoroscopy: computer-assisted fluoroscopic navigation*, Spine, 26 (2001), pp. 347–351.

[64] E. FRITSCH, *Navigation in spinal surgery using fluoroscopy*, in Navigation and Robotics in Total Joint and Spine Surgery, J. B. Stiehl, W. H. Konermann, and R. G. A. Haaker, eds., Springer, 2004, ch. 68, pp. 487–494.

[65] D. FRYBACK AND J. THORNBURY, *The efficacy of diagnostic imaging*, Medical Decision Making, 11 (1991), p. 88.

[66] H. FUCHS, M. A. LIVINGSTON, R. RASKAR, D. COLUCCI, K. KELLER, A. STATE, J. R. CRAWFORD, P. RADEMACHER, S. H. DRAKE, AND A. A. MEYER, *Augmented reality visualization for laparoscopic surgery*, in Proceedings of the First International Conference of Medical Image Computing and Computer-Assisted Intervention (MICCAI), I. W. M. Wells, A. C. F. Colchester, and S. L. Delp, eds., vol. 1496 of Lecture Notes in Computer Science, Cambridge, MA, USA, October 1998, Springer-Verlag, pp. 934–943.

[67] R. GALLOWAY, *The process and development of image-guided procedures*, Annual Review of Biomedical Engineering, 3 (2001), pp. 83–108.

[68] R. GALLOWAY AND T. PETERS, *Overview and History of Image-Guided Interventions*, Image-Guided Interventions - Technology and Applications, Springer, 2008, ch. 1.

[69] F. GEBHARD, L. KINZL, AND M. ARAND, *Grenzen der CT-basierten Computernavigation in der Wirbelsäulenchirurgie*, Der Unfallchirurg, 103 (2000), pp. 696–701.

[70] F. GEBHARD, M. K. E. SCHNEIDER, M. ARAND, L. KINZL, A. HEBECKER, AND L. BÄTZ, *Radiation dosage in orthopedics - a comparison of computer-assisted procedures*, Unfallchirurg, 106(6) (2003), pp. 492–497.

[71] J. GEERLING, U. BERLEMANN, B. FRERICKS, M. KFURI, T. HÜFNER, AND C. KRETTEK, *Pedicle screw placement*, in Navigation and Robotics in Total Joint and Spine Surgery, J. B. Stiehl, W. H. Konermann, and R. G. A. Haaker, eds., Springer, 2004, ch. 67, pp. 481–486.

[72] H. GEIJER, K.-W. BECKMAN, B. JONSSON, T. ANDERSSON, AND J. PERSLIDEN, *Digital radiography of scoliosis with a scanning method: Initial evaluation*, Radiology, 218: (2001), pp. 402–410.

[73] P. L. GILDENBERG, *The History of Stereotactic and Functional Neurosurgery*, Textbook of Stereotactic and Functional Neurosurgery, McGraw-Hill, 1998, ch. 1, pp. 5–19.

[74] P. L. GILDENBERG AND R. R. TASKER, eds., *Textbook of Stereotactic and Functional Neurosurgery*, McGraw-Hill, 1998.

[75] F. GIRARDI, F. CAMMISA, H. SANDHU, AND L. ALVAREZ, *The placement of lumbar pedicle screws using computerised stereotactic guidance*, Journal of Bone & Joint Surgery, British Volume, 81 (1999), pp. 825–829.

[76] S. GOLD AND A. RANGARAJAN, *A graduated assignment algorithm for graph matching*, IEEE Trans. Pattern Anal. Machine Intell., 18 (1996), pp. 377–388.

[77] C. S. GOODMAN, *Introduction to health care technology assessment*. Online, 1998. Nat. Library Medicine/NICHSR.

[78] W. GRIMSON, G. ETTINGER, S. WHITE, T. LOZANO-PEREZ, W. WELLS III, AND R. KIKINIS, *An automatic registration method for frameless stereotaxy, imageguided surgery, and enhanced reality visualization*, Medical Imaging, IEEE Transactions on, 15 (1996), pp. 129–140.

[79] P. A. GRÜTZNER, A. HEBECKER, H. WAELTI, B. VOCK, L.-P. NOLTE, AND A. WENTZENSEN, *Clinical study for registration-free 3d-navigation with the siremobil iso-c^{3D} mobile c-arm*, electromedica, 71 (2003), pp. 7–16.

References

[80] M. HADWIGER, J. M. KNISS, C. REZK-SALAMA, AND D. WEISKOPF, *Real-time Volume Graphics*, A K Peters, 2006.

[81] J. HAJNAL, D. HAWKES, AND D. HILL, *Medical Image Registration*, CRC Press, 2001.

[82] R. A. HART, B. L. HANSEN, M. SHEA, F. HSU, AND G. J. ANDERSON, *Pedicle screw placement in the thoracic spine: a comparison of image-guided and manual techniques in cadavers*, Spine., 30 (2005), pp. 326–331.

[83] R. HARTLEY AND A. ZISSERMAN, *Multiple View Geometry in Computer Vision*, Cambridge University Press, 2nd ed., 2003.

[84] D. HAWKES, D. BARRATT, T. CARTER, J. MCCLELLAND, AND B. CRUM, *Non-Rigid Registration*, Image-Guided Interventions - Technology and Applications, Springer, 2008, ch. 7.

[85] M. HAYASHIBE, N. SUZUKI, A. HATTORI, Y. OTAKE, S. SUZUKI, AND N. NAKATA, *Surgical navigation display system using volume rendering of intraoperatively scanned ct images*, Computer Aided Surgery, 11 (2006), pp. 240–246.

[86] J. HEIKKILÄ AND O. SILVÉN, *A four-step camera calibration procedure with implicit image correction*, in Proc. IEEE Conf. Computer Vision and Pattern Recognition (CVPR), IEEE Computer Society, 1997, pp. 1106–1112.

[87] S. HEINING, E. EULER, S. WIESNER, AND N. NAVAB, *Pedicle screw placement under video-augmented fluoroscopic control: First clinical application - a cadaver study*, in CARS 2006 - Computer Assisted Radiology and Surgery, June 2006.

[88] S.-M. HEINING, P. STEFAN, L. OMARY, S. WIESNER, T. SIELHORST, N. NAVAB, F. SAUER, E. EULER, W. MUTSCHLER, AND J. TRAUB, *Evaluation of an insitu visualization system for navigated trauma surgery*, Journal of Biomechanics, 39 (2006), p. 209.

[89] S.-M. HEINING, S. WIESNER, E. EULER, W. MUTSCHLER, AND N. NAVAB, *Locking of intramedullary nails under video-augmented flouroscopic control: first clinical application in a cadaver study*, in Proceedings of The 6th Computer Assisted Orthopaedic Surgery (CAOS 2006), Montreal, Canada, June 2006.

[90] W. R. HENDEE AND E. R. RITENOUR, *Medical Imaging Physics*, John Wiley & Sons Inc, 4th ed., 2002.

[91] W. HOFF, *Fusion of data from head-mounted and fixed sensors*, in Proceedings of First International Workshop on Augmented Reality IWAR, 1998.

[92] W. A. HOFF AND T. L. VINCENT, *Analysis of head pose accuracy in augmented reality*, IEEE Trans. Visualization and Computer Graphics, 6 (2000).

References

[93] E. J. HOFFMAN, M. P. TORNAI, M. JANECEK, B. E. PATT, AND J. S. IWANCZYK, *Intraoperative probes and imaging probes*, European Journal of Nuclear Medicine and Molecular Imaging, 26 (1999), pp. 913–935.

[94] C. HOHL, J. BÖSE, T. BRUNNER, R. BANCKWITZ, G. MÜHLENBRUCH, J. WILDBERGER, A. MAHNKEN, AND R. GÜNTHER, *Angiographische ct: Messung der effektiven patientendosis*, in 88. Deutscher Röntgenkongress, 2007.

[95] R. HOLLOWAY, *Registration error analysis for augmented reality*, Presence: Teleoperators and Virtual Env., 6 (1997), pp. 413–432.

[96] L. HOLLY AND K. FOLEY, *Intraoperative spinal navigation*, Spine, 28 (2003), pp. 554–561.

[97] L. T. HOLLY, *Image-guided spinal surgery*, The International Journal of Medical Robotics and Computer Assisted Surgery, 2 (2006), pp. 7–15.

[98] V. HORSLEY AND R. CLARKE, *The structure and functions of the cerebellum examined by a new method*, Brain, 31 (1908), pp. 45–124.

[99] J. HUMMEL, M. FIGL, W. BIRKFELLNER, M. R. BAX, R. SHAHIDI, C. R. MAURER, JR., AND H. BERGMANN, *Evaluation of a new electromagnetic tracking system using a standardized assessment protocol*, Physics in Medicine and Biology, 51 (2006), pp. 205–210.

[100] J. HUMMEL, M.FIGL, W. BIRKFELLNER, C. KOLLMANN, AND H.BERGMANN, *Evaluation of an electromagnetic tracking system*, Medical Physics, 29 (2002), pp. 2205–2212.

[101] J. B. HUMMEL, M. R. BAX, M. L. FIGL, Y. KANG, C. MAURER, JR., W. W. BIRKFELLNER, H. BERGMANN, AND R. SHAHIDI, *Design and application of an assessment protocol for electromagnetic tracking systems*, Medical Physics, 32 (2005), pp. 2371–2379.

[102] INTERNATIONAL ORGANIZATION FOR STANDARDIZATION, *Iso 9000:2005 quality management systems - fundamentals and vocabulary*.

[103] I. JACOBSON, G. BOOCH, AND J. RUMBAUGH, *Unified Software Development Process*, Addison-Wesley Longman, Amsterdam, 1999.

[104] P. JANNIN, J. FITZPATRICK, D. HAWKES, X. PENNEC, R. SHAHIDI, AND M. VANNIER, *Validation of medical image processing in image-guided therapy*, IEEE Trans. Med. Imag., 21 (2002), pp. 1445–1449.

[105] P. JANNIN, C. GROVA, AND C. R. MAURER, *Model for defining and reporting reference-based validation protocols in medical image processing*, International Journal of Computer Assisted Radiology and Surgery, 1 (2006), pp. 63–73.

References

[106] P. JANNIN AND W. KORB, *Image-Guided Interventions - Technology and Applications*, vol. chapter 18, Springer, May 2008.

[107] P. JANNIN AND X. MORANDI, *Surgical models for computer-assisted neurosurgery*, NeuroImage, 37 (2007), pp. 783–791.

[108] P. JANNIN, M. RAIMBAULT, X. MORANDI, AND B. GIBAUD, *Modeling surgical procedures for multimodal image-guided neurosurgery*, in Proc. Int'l Conf. Medical Image Computing and Computer Assisted Intervention (MICCAI), vol. 2208 of Lecture Notes in Computer Science, Springer-Verlag, 2001, pp. 565–572.

[109] P. JANNIN, M. RAIMBAULT, X. MORANDI, E. SEIGNEURET, AND B. GIBAUD, *Design of a neurosurgical procedure model for multimodal image-guided surgery*, in CARS 2001 - Computer Assisted Radiology and Surgery, 2001, pp. 102–106.

[110] B. JARAMAZ AND I. A. M. DIGIOIA, *Ct-based navigation systems*, in Navigation and Robotics in Total Joint and Spine Surgery, J. B. Stiehl, W. H. Konermann, and R. G. A. Haaker, eds., Springer, 2003, ch. 2, pp. 10–16.

[111] I. KALFAS, D. KORMOS, M. MURPHY, R. MCKENZIE, G. BARNETT, G. BELL, C. STEINER, M. TRIMBLE, AND J. WEISENBERGER, *Application of frameless stereotaxy to pedicle screw fixation of the spine*, Journal of neurosurgery, 83 (1995), pp. 641–647.

[112] M. KAMIMURA, S. EBARA, H. ITOH, Y. TATEIWA, T. KINOSHITA, AND K. TAKAOKA, *Accurate pedicle screw insertion under the control of a computer-assisted image guiding system: Laboratory test and clinical study*, Journal of Orthopaedic Science, 4 (1999), pp. 197–206.

[113] M. KASS, A. WITKIN, AND D. TERZOPOULOS, *Snakes: Active contour models*, Int'l J. of Comp. Vision, 1 (1988), pp. 321–331.

[114] P. J. KELLY, G. ALKER, AND S. GOERSS, *Computer-assisted stereotactic laser microsurgery for the treatment of intracranial neoplasms*, Neurosurgery, 10 (1982), pp. 324–331.

[115] R. KHADEM, C. C. YEH, M. SADEGHI-TEHRANI, M. R. BAX, J. A. JOHNSON, J. N. WELCH, E. P. WILKINSON, AND R. SHAHIDI, *Comparative tracking error analysis of five different optical tracking systems*, Computer Aided Surgery, 5 (2000), pp. 98–107.

[116] V. V. KINDRATENKO, *A survey of electromagnetic position tracker calibration techniques*, Virtual Reality: Research, Development, and Applications, 5 (2000), pp. 169–182.

[117] A. P. KING, P. J. EDWARDS, C. R. MAURER, JR., D. A. DE CUNHA, D. J. HAWKES, D. L. G. HILL, R. P. GASTON, M. R. FENLON, A. J. STRONG, C. L. CHANDLER, A. RICHARDS, AND M. J. GLEESON, *Design and evaluation of a*

system for microscope-assisted guided interventions, IEEE Trans. Med. Imag., 19 (2000), pp. 1082–1093.

[118] T. KLEIN, J. TRAUB, H. HAUTMANN, A. AHMADIAN, AND N. NAVAB, *Fiducial free registration procedure for navigated bronchoscopy*, in In Proceedings of Medical Image Computing and Computer Assisted Intervention (MICCAI), 2007, pp. 475–482.

[119] C. KNOP, M.BLAUTH, L. BASTIAN, U. LANGE, J. KESTING, AND H. TSCHERNE, *Frakturen der thorakolumbalen wirbelsäule - spätergebnisse nach dorsaler instrumentierung und ihre konsequenzen*, Unfallchirurg, 100 (1997), pp. 630–639.

[120] R. KOPPE, E. KLOTZ, J. DE BEEK, AND H. AERTS, *3D vessel reconstruction based on rotational angiography*, in Proceedings of Computer Assisted Radiology (CAR Š95), 1995, pp. 101–107.

[121] W. KORB, R. GRUNERT, O. BURGERT, H. LEMKE, A. DIETZ, V. FALK, S. JACOBS, J. MEIXENSBERGER, G. STRAUSS, C. TRANTAKIS, AND P. JANNIN, *An assessment model of the efficacy of image guided therapy*, in Computer Assisted Radiology and Surgery, 2006.

[122] Y. KOTANI, K. ABUMI, M. ITO, M. TAKAHATA, H. SUDO, S. OHSHIMA, AND A. MINAMI, *Accuracy analysis of pedicle screw placement in posterior scoliosis surgery: Comparison between conventional fluoroscopic and computer-assisted technique*, Spine, 32 (2007), pp. 1543–1550.

[123] A. KRIEGER, R. SUSIL, C. MENARD, J. COLEMAN, G. FICHTINGER, E. ATALAR, AND L. WHITCOMB, *Design of a novel MRI compatible manipulator for image guided prostate interventions*, Biomedical Engineering, IEEE Transactions on, 52 (2005), pp. 306–313.

[124] J. KRÜGER, J. SCHNEIDER, AND R. WESTERMANN, *ClearView: An interactive context preserving hotspot visualization technique*, IEEE Transactions on Visualization and Computer Graphics (Proceedings Visualization / Information Visualization 2006), 12 (2006), pp. 941–948.

[125] W. LAI AND H. DUH, *Effects of frame rate for visualization of dynamic quantitative information in a head-mounted display*, in Systems, Man and Cybernetics, 2004 IEEE International Conference on, vol. 7, 2004.

[126] T. LAINE, T. LUND, M. YLIKOSKI, J. LOHIKOSKI, AND D. SCHLENZKA, *Accuracy of pedicle screw insertion with and without computer assistance: a randomised controlled clinical study in 100 consecutive patients*, European Spine Journal, 9 (2000), pp. 235–240.

[127] T. LAINE, D. SCHLENZKA, K. MAKITALO, K. TALLROTH, L. NOLTE, AND H. VISARIUS, *Improved accuracy of pedicle screw insertion with computer-assisted surgery. a prospective clinical trial of 30 patients*, Spine, 22 (1997), pp. 1254–1258.

References

[128] F. LANGLOTZ AND E. KEEVE, *Minimally invasive approaches in orthopaedic surgery*, Minimally Invasive Therapy and Allied Technologies, 12 (2003), pp. 19–24.

[129] F. LANGLOTZ AND L. NOLTE, *Computer-assisted minimally invasive spine surgery - state of the art*, in Minimally Invasive Spine Surgery - A Surgical Manual, H. M. Mayer, ed., Springer, 2006, ch. 6, pp. 26–32.

[130] W. LAU, *History of Endoscopic and Laparoscopic Surgery*, World Journal of Surgery, 21 (1997), pp. 444–453.

[131] S. LAVEALLE, G. C. BURDEA, AND R. TAYLOR, eds., *Computer-Integrated Surgery: Technology and Clinical Applications*, MIT Press, 1996.

[132] H. U. LEMKE, *Summary of the white paper of dicom wg24 'dicom in surgery'*, in Proceedings of the SPIE Medical Imaging 2007: PACS and Imaging Informatics., S. C. Horii and K. P. Andriole, eds., vol. 6516 of Proceedings of SPIE, March 2007.

[133] H. U. LEMKE AND L. BERLINER, *Specification and design of a therapy imaging and model management system (timms)*, in Proceedings of the SPIE Medical Imaging 2007: PACS and Imaging Informatics., S. C. Horii and K. P. Andriole, eds., vol. 6516 of Presented at the Society of Photo-Optical Instrumentation Engineers (SPIE) Conference, March 2007, pp. 651–602.

[134] H. U. LEMKE AND M. W. VANNIER, *The operating room and the need for an it infrastructure and standards*, International Journal of Computer Assisted Radiology and Surgery, 1 (2006), pp. 117–121.

[135] J. LEVEN, D. BURSCHKA, R. KUMAR, G. ZHANG, S. BLUMENKRANZ, X. D. DAI, M. AWAD, G. D. HAGER, M. MAROHN, M. CHOTI, C. HASSER, AND R. H. TAYLOR, *Davinci canvas: A telerobotic surgical system with integrated, robot-assisted, laparoscopic ultrasound capability*, in Proc. Int'l Conf. Medical Image Computing and Computer Assisted Intervention (MICCAI), vol. 3749 of Lecture Notes in Computer Science, Springer-Verlag, September 2005, pp. 811–818.

[136] H. LIN, I. SHAFRAN, D. YUH, AND G. HAGER, *Towards automatic skill evaluation: Detection and segmentation of robot-assisted surgical motions*, Computer Aided Surgery, 11 (2006), pp. 220–230.

[137] G. LITYNSKI, *Endoscopic Surgery: The History, the Pioneers*, World Journal of Surgery, 23 (1999), pp. 745–753.

[138] H. LIU, Y. YU, M. C. SCHELL, W. G. O'DELL, R. RUO, AND P. OKUNIEFF, *Optimal marker placement in photogrammetry patient positioning system*, Medical Physics, 30 (2003), pp. 103–110.

[139] M. A. LIVINGSTON AND A. STATE, *Magnetic tracker calibration for improved augmented reality registration*, Presence: Teleoperators and Virtual Env., 6 (1997), pp. 532–546.

[140] H. LIVYATAN, Z. YANIV, AND L. JOSKOWICZ, *Robust automatic c-arm calibration for fluoroscopy-based navigation: A practical approach*, in Proceedings of Medical Image Computing and Computer-Assisted Intervention (Miccai), vol. 2489, Springer, 2002, pp. 60–68.

[141] B. P. L. LO, A. DARZI, AND G.-Z. YANG, *Episode classification for the analysis of tissue/instrument interaction with multiple visual cues*, in Proceedings of Medical Image Computing and Computer Assisted Interventions (MICCAI), 2003, pp. 230–237.

[142] M. H. LOSER AND N. NAVAB, *A new robotic system for visually controlled percutaneous interventions under ct fluoroscopy*, in Proceedings of Medical Image Computing and Computer Assisted Interventions (MICCAI), 2000.

[143] C. P. LU, G. D. HAGER, AND E. MJOLSNESS, *Fast and globally convergent pose estimation from video images*, IEEE Trans. Pattern Anal. Machine Intell., 22 (2000), pp. 610–622.

[144] J. B. A. MAINTZ AND M. A. VIERGEVER, *A survey of medical image registration*, Medical Image Analysis, 2 (1998), pp. 1–36.

[145] B. MANSOUX, L. NIGAY, AND J. TROCCAZ, *Interaction between a surgeon and a computer assisted surgery system: an interactive design space*, in Proceedings of SURGETICA, Chambery, France, 2005.

[146] K. MASAMUNE, G. FICHTINGER, A. DEGUET, D. MATSUKA, AND R. TAYLOR, *An image overlay system with enhanced reality for percutaneous therapy performed inside ct scanner*, in Proc. Int'l Conf. Medical Image Computing and Computer Assisted Intervention (MICCAI), 2002.

[147] J. M. MATHIS, ed., *Image-Guided Spine Interventions*, Springer, 2004.

[148] J. M. MATHIS, H. DERAMOND, AND S. M. BELKOFF, eds., *Percutaneous Vertebroplasty and Kyphoplasty*, Springer, 2nd ed., 2006.

[149] H. M. MAYER, *Minimally invasive spine surgery*, in Minimally Invasive Spine Surgery - A Surgical Manual, H. M. Mayer, ed., Springer, 2006, ch. 1, pp. 3–7.

[150] H. M. MAYER, *Minimally Invasive Spine Surgery*, Springer, 2006.

[151] G. MEGALI, S. SINIGAGLIA, O. TONET, AND P. DARIO, *Modelling and evaluation of surgical performance using hidden markov models*, Biomedical Engineering, IEEE Transactions on, 53 (2006), pp. 1911–1919.

[152] P. MERLOZ, S. LAVALLEE, C. HUBERSON, I. TONETTI, L. PITTET, A. EID, S. PLAWESKI, T. MARTINEZ, P. CINQUIN, AND J. TROCCAZ, *Computerised pedicular screw fixation: technology and clinical practice*, vol. Surgical Techniques in Orthopaedics and Traumatology (v. 2): Spine, Elsevier, 2003, ch. 5, pp. 37–46.

References

[153] P. MERLOZ, J. TONETTI, L. PITTET, M. COULOMB, S. LAVALLEE, AND P. SAUTOT, *Pedicle screw placement using image guided techniques*, Clin Orthop Relat Res, 354 (1998), pp. 39–48.

[154] P. MESSMER, F. MATTHEWS, C. WULLSCHLEGER, R. HÜGLI, P. REGAZZONI, AND A. L. JACOB, *Image fusion for intraoperative control of axis in long bone fracture treatment*, European Journal of Trauma, Volume 32, Number 6 (December, 2006), pp. 555–561.

[155] M. MITSCHKE, A. BANI-HASHEMI, AND N. NAVAB, *Interventions under video-augmented x-ray guidance: Application to needle placement*, in Proc. Int'l Conf. Medical Image Computing and Computer Assisted Intervention (MICCAI), vol. 1935 of Lecture Notes in Computer Science, Springer-Verlag, October 2000, pp. 858–868.

[156] M. MITSCHKE AND N. NAVAB, *Recovering projection geometry: How a cheap camera can outperform an expensive stereo system*, in Proc. IEEE Conf. Computer Vision and Pattern Recognition (CVPR), vol. 1, 2000, pp. 193–200.

[157] ——, *Recovering x-ray projection geometry for 3d tomographic reconstruction: Use of integrated camera vs. external navigation system*, International Journal of Medical Image Analysis (MIA), 7 (2003), pp. 65–78.

[158] M. MOGHARI AND P. ABOLMAESUMI, *A novel incremental technique for ultrasound to ct bone surface registration using unscented kalman filtering*, in Proceedings of Medical Image Computing and Computer Assisted Interventions (MICCAI 2005), Springer, 2005, pp. 197–204.

[159] K. MORI, D. DEGUCHI, K. AKIYAMA, T. KITASAKA, C. R. MAURER, JR., Y. SUENAGA, H. TAKABATAKE, M. MORI, , AND H. NATORI, *Hybrid bronchoscope tracking using a magnetic tracking sensor and image registration*, in Proc. Int'l Conf. Medical Image Computing and Computer Assisted Intervention (MICCAI), Springer-Verlag, 2005, pp. 543–550.

[160] D. MUCHA, B. KOSMECKI, AND J. BIER, *Plausibility check for error compensation in electromagnetic navigation in endoscopic sinus surgery*, International Journal of Computer Assisted Radiology and Surgery, 1 (2006), pp. 316–318.

[161] C. NAFIS, V. JENSEN, L. BEAUREGARD, AND P. ANDERSON, *Method for estimating dynamic em tracking accuracy of surgical navigation tools*, in Medical Imaging 2006: Visualization, Image-Guided Procedures, and Display, K. R. Cleary and R. L. Galloway, Jr., eds., vol. 6141 of Proceedings of SPIE, March 2006.

[162] M. NAKAMOTO, Y. SATO, M. MIYAMOTO, Y. NAKAMJIMA, K. KONISHI, M. SHIMADA, M. HASHIZUME, AND S. TAMURA, *3d ultrasound system using a magneto-optic hybrid tracker for augmented reality visualization in laparoscopic liver surgery*, in Proc. Int'l Conf. Medical Image Computing and Computer Assisted Intervention

References

(MICCAI), T. Dohi and R. Kikinis, eds., vol. 2489 of Lecture Notes in Computer Science, Springer-Verlag, 2002, pp. 148–155.

[163] N. NAVAB, A. BANI-HASHEMI, M. S. NADAR, K. WIESENT, P. DURLAK, T. BRUNNER, K. BARTH, AND R. GRAUMANN, *3d reconstruction from projection matrices in a c-arm based 3d-angiography system*, in Proceedings of the First International Conference of Medical Image Computing and Computer-Assisted Intervention (MICCAI), I. W. M. Wells, A. C. F. Colchester, and S. L. Delp, eds., vol. 1496 of Lecture Notes in Computer Science, Cambridge, MA, USA, October 1998, pp. 119–129.

[164] N. NAVAB, A. R. BANI-HASHEMI, M. M. MITSCHKE, D. W. HOLDSWORTH, R. FAHRIG, A. J. FOX, AND R. GRAUMANN, *Dynamic geometrical calibration for 3d cerebral angiography*, in Medical Imaging 1996: Physics of Medical Imaging, vol. 2708 of Proceedings of SPIE, 1996, pp. 361–370.

[165] N. NAVAB, M. FEUERSTEIN, AND C. BICHLMEIER, *Laparoscopic virtual mirror - new interaction paradigm for monitor based augmented reality*, in Virtual Reality, Charlotte, North Carolina, USA, March 2007, pp. 43–50.

[166] N. NAVAB AND M. MITSCHKE, *Method and apparatus using a virtual detector for three-dimensional reconstruction form x-ray images.* Patent US 6236704; Filing date: Jun 30, 1999; Issue date: May 22, 2001, 1999.

[167] N. NAVAB, M. MITSCHKE, AND A. BANI-HASHEMI, *Merging visible and invisible: Two camera-augmented mobile C-arm (CAMC) applications*, in Proc. IEEE and ACM Int'l Workshop on Augmented Reality, San Francisco, CA, USA, 1999, pp. 134–141.

[168] N. NAVAB, M. MITSCHKE, AND O. SCHÜTZ, *Camera-augmented mobile c-arm (camc) application: 3d reconstruction using a low-cost mobile c-arm*, in Proc. Int'l Conf. Medical Image Computing and Computer Assisted Intervention (MICCAI), C. Taylor and A. Colchester, eds., vol. 1679 of Lecture Notes in Computer Science, Springer-Verlag, 1999, pp. 688–697.

[169] N. NAVAB, J. TRAUB, T. SIELHORST, M. FEUERSTEIN, AND C. BICHLMEIER, *Action- and workflow-driven augmented reality for computer-aided medical procedures*, IEEE Computer Graphics and Applications, 27 (2007), pp. 10–14.

[170] N. NAVAB, J. TRAUB, T. WENDLER, A. BUCK, AND S. I. ZIEGLER, *Navigated nuclear probes for intra-operative functional imaging*, in Proceedings of the 5th IEEE International Symposium on Biomedical Imaging: From Nano to Macro (to appear), 2008.

[171] N. NAVAB, S. WIESNER, S. BENHIMANE, E. EULER, AND S. M. HEINING, *Visual servoing for intraoperative positioning and repositioning of mobile c-arms*, in Proc. Int'l Conf. Medical Image Computing and Computer Assisted Intervention (MICCAI), 2006.

References

[172] T. NEUMUTH, N. DURSTEWITZ, M. FISCHER, G. STRAUSS, A. DIETZ, J. MEIXENSBERGER, P. JANNIN, K. CLEARY, H. U. LEMKE, AND O. BURGERT, *Structured recording of intraoperative surgical workflows,*, in SPIE Medical Imaging - 2006 - PACS and Imaging Informatics - 61450A, vol. 7 of Progress in Biomedical Optics and Imaging, The International Society for Optical Engeneering, 2006.

[173] T. NEUMUTH, S. SCHUMANN, G. STRAUSS, P. JANNIN, J. MEIXENSBERGER, A. DIETZ, H. U. LEMKE, AND O. BURGERT, *Visualization options for surgical workflows*, International Journal of Computer Assisted Radiology and Surgery, 1 (2006), pp. 438–440.

[174] W. NIESSEN, *Model-based Image Segmentation for Image-Guided Interventions*, Image-Guided Interventions - Technology and Applications, Springer, 2008, ch. 8.

[175] L. NOLTE, M. SLOMCZYKOWSKI, U. BERLEMANN, M. STRAUSS, R. HOFSTETTER, D. SCHLENZKA, T. LAINE, AND T. LUND, *A new approach to computer-aided spine surgery: fluoroscopy-based surgical navigation*, European Spine Journal, 9 (2000), pp. 78–88.

[176] L.-P. NOLTE AND F. LANGLOTZ, *Basics of computer-assisted orthopaedic surgery (caos)*, in Navigation and Robotics in Total Joint and Spine Surgery, J. B. Stiehl, W. H. Konermann, and R. G. A. Haaker, eds., Springer, 2004, ch. 1, pp. 3–9.

[177] L. P. NOLTE, L. J. ZAMORANO, Z. JIANG, Q. WANG, F. LANGLOTZ, AND U. BERLEMANN, *Image-guided insertion of transpedicular screws. a laboratory set-up*, Spine., 20 (1995), pp. 497–500.

[178] S. OSHER AND J. A. SETHIAN, *Fronts propagating with curvature dependent speed: Algorithms based on Hamilton-Jacobi formulations*, J. Computational Physics, 79 (1988), pp. 12–49.

[179] N. PADOY, T. BLUM, I. ESSA, H. FEUSSNER, M.-O. BERGER, AND N. NAVAB, *A boosted segmentation method for surgical workflow analysis*, in International Conference on Medical Image Computing and Computer-Assisted Intervention (MICCAI), Brisbane, Australia, October 2007.

[180] N. PADOY, T. BLUM, H. FEUSSNER, M. BERGER, AND N. NAVAB, *On-line recognition of surgical activity for monitoring in the operating room*, in Proceedings of the 20th Conference on Innovative Applications of Artificial Intelligence (IAAI-08), 2008.

[181] N. PADOY, T. BLUM, H. FEUSSNER, M.-O. BERGER, AND N. NAVAB, *On-line recognition of surgical activity for monitoring in the operating room*, (2008).

[182] B. PATT, M. TORNAI, J. IWANCZYK, C. LEVIN, AND E. HOFFMAN, *Development of an intraoperative gamma camera based on a 256-pixel mercuric iodide detector array*, IEEE Trans. Nucl. Sci., 44 (1997), pp. 1242–1248.

[183] T. PETERS, *Image-guidance for surgical procedures*, Physics in Medicine and Biology, 51 (2006), pp. R505–R540.

[184] T. PETERS AND K. CLEARY, eds., *Image-Guided Interventions - Technology and Applications*, Springer, May 2008.

[185] T. M. PETERS, *Image-guided surgery: From x-rays to virtual reality*, Computer Methods in Biomechanics and Biomedical Engineering, (2000).

[186] D. L. PHAM, C. XU, AND J. L. PRINCE, *Current methods in medical image segmentation*, Annual Review of Biomedical Engineering, 2 (2000), pp. 315–337.

[187] M. E. P. PHELPS, E. HOFFMAN, N. MULLANI, AND M. TER-POGOSSIAN, *Application of annihilation coincidence detection to transaxial reconstruction tomography*, J Nucl Med., 16 (1975), pp. 210—224.

[188] F. RAAB, E. BLOOD, T. STEIONER, AND H. JONES, *Magnetic position and orientation tracking system*, IEEE Transactions on Aerospace and Electronic Systems, 15 (1979), pp. 709–718.

[189] S. RAJASEKARAN, S. VIDYADHARA, P. RAMESH, AND A. P. SHETTY, *Randomized clinical study to compare the accuracy of navigated and non-navigated thoracic pedicle screws in deformity correction surgeries*, Spine, 32 (2007), pp. E56–E64.

[190] Y. R. RAMPERSAUD, K. T. FOLEY, A. C. SHEN, S. WILLIAMS, AND M. SOLOMITO, *Radiation exposure to the spine surgeon during fluoroscopically assisted pedicle screw insertion.*, Spine., 25 (2000), pp. 2637–2645.

[191] D. K. RESNICK AND S. R. GARFIN, eds., *Vertebroplasty and Kyphoplasty*, Thieme Medical Publishers, 2005.

[192] D. RITTER, M. MITSCHKE, AND R. GRAUMANN, *Markerless navigation with the intra-operative imaging modality siremobil iso-c^{3D}*, electromedica, 70 (2002), pp. 31–36.

[193] D. ROBERTS, J. STROHBEHN, J. HATCH, W. MURRAY, AND H. KETTENBERGER, *A frameless stereotaxic integration of computerized tomographic imaging and the operating microscope.*, J Neurosurg, 65 (1986), pp. 545–9.

[194] K. ROESSLER, K. UNGERSBOECK, W. DIETRICH, M. AICHHOLZER, K. HITTMEIR, C. MATULA, T. CZECH, AND W. KOOS, *Frameless stereotactic guided neurosurgery: clinical experience with an infrared based pointer device navigation system*, Acta Neurochir, 139 (1997), pp. 551–955.

[195] J. ROLLAND, L. DAVIS, AND Y. BAILLOT, *A survey of tracking technology for virtual environments*, 2001, pp. 67–112.

References

[196] J. ROSEN, J. BROWN, L. CHANG, M. SINANAN, AND B. HANNAFORD, *Generalized approach for modeling minimally invasive surgery as a stochastic process using a discrete markov model*, Biomedical Engineering, IEEE Transactions on, 53 (2006), pp. 399–413.

[197] J. ROSEN, B. HANNAFORD, C. RICHARDS, AND M. SINANAN, *Markov modeling of minimally invasive surgery based on tool/tissueinteraction and force/torque signatures for evaluating surgical skills*, Biomedical Engineering, IEEE Transactions on, 48 (2001), pp. 579–591.

[198] M. ROSENTHAL, A. STATE, J. LEE, G. HIROTA, J. ACKERMAN, E. D. P. KURTIS KELLER, M. JIROUTEK, K. MULLER, AND H. FUCHS, *Augmented reality guidance for needle biopsies: An initial randomized, controlled trial in phantoms*, Medical Image Analysis, 6 (2002), pp. 313–320.

[199] A. ROUGEE, C. PICARD, C. PONCHUT, AND Y. TROUSSET, *Geometrical calibration of X-ray imaging chains for three-dimensional reconstruction.*, Comput Med Imaging Graph, 17 (1993), pp. 295–300.

[200] R.RAO AND M. SINGRAKHIA, *Fundamentals in Spine Surgery*, Springer, 2004, ch. 65, pp. 467–476.

[201] J. RUMBAUGH, I. JACOBSON, AND G. BOOCH, *The Unified Modeling Language Reference Manual*, Addison-Wesley Longman, Amsterdam, 2nd ed., 2004.

[202] F. SAUER, A. KHAMENE, B. BASCLE, AND G. J. RUBINO, *A head-mounted display system for augmented reality image guidance: Towards clinical evaluation for imriguided neurosurgery*, in Proc. Int'l Conf. Medical Image Computing and Computer Assisted Intervention (MICCAI), London, UK, 2001, Springer-Verlag, pp. 707–716.

[203] F. SAUER, A. KHAMENE, B. BASCLE, L. SCHIMMANG, F. WENZEL, , AND S. VOGT, *Augmented reality visualization of ultrasound images: systemdescription, calibration, and features*, in Proc. IEEE and ACM Int'l Symp. on Augmented Reality, 2001, pp. 30–39.

[204] F. SAUER, U. J. SCHOEPF, A. KHAMENE, S. VOGT, M. DAS, AND S. G. SILVERMAN, *Augmented reality system for ct-guided interventions: System description and initial phantom trials*, in Medical Imaging: Visualization, Image-Guided Procedures, and Display, 2003.

[205] F. SAUER, S. VOGT, AND A. KHAMENE, *Augmented Reality*, Image-Guided Interventions - Technology and Applications, Springer, 2008, ch. 4.

[206] F. SAUER, F. WENZEL, S. VOGT, Y. TAO, Y. GENC, AND A. BANI-HASHEMI, *Augmented workspace: designing an ar testbed*, in Proc. IEEE and ACM Int'l Symp. on Augmented Reality, 2000, pp. 47–53.

[207] K. SCHICHO, M. FIGL, M. DONAT, W. BIRKFELLNER, R. SEEMANN, A. WAGNER, H. BERGMANN, AND R. EWERS, *Stability of miniature electromagnetic tracking systems*, Physics in Medicine and Biology, 50 (2005), pp. 2089–2098.

[208] C. SCHULZE, E. MUNZINGER, U. WEBER, AND S. GERTZBEIN, *Clinical relevance of accuracy of pedicle screw placement: A computed tomographic-supported analysis. Point of view*, Spine(Philadelphia, PA. 1976), 23 (1998), pp. 2215–2221.

[209] O. SCHWARZENBACH, U. BERLEMANN, B. JOST, H. VISARIUS, E. ARM, F. LANGLOTZ, L. NOLTE, AND C. OZDOBA, *Accuracy of computer-assisted pedicle screw placement. An in vivo computed tomography analysis*, Spine, 22 (1997), pp. 452–458.

[210] J. G. SEMPLE AND G. T. KNEEBONE, *Algebraic Projective Geometry*, Oxford University Press, USA, 1998.

[211] J. A. SETHIAN, *Level Set Methods and Fast Marching Methods. Evolving Interfaces in Computational Geometry, Fluid Mechanics, Computer Vision, and Materials Science*, no. 3 in Cambridge Monographs on Applied and Computational Mathematics, Cambridge University Press, 2nd ed., 1999.

[212] K. SHAH AND R. WEISSLEDER, *Molecular optical imaging: applications leading to the development of present day therapeutics.*, NeuroRx, 2 (2005), pp. 215–225.

[213] R. SHAHIDI, M. R. BAX, C. R. MAURER, JR., J. A. JOHNSON, E. P. WILKINSON, B. WANG, J. B. WEST, M. J. CITARDI, K. H. MANWARING, AND R. KHADEM, *Implementation, calibration and accuracy testing of an image-enhanced endoscopy system*, IEEE Trans. Med. Imag., 21 (2002), pp. 1524–1535.

[214] T. SIELHORST, *New Methods for Medical Augmented Reality*, PhD thesis, Technische Universität München (TUM), Chair for Computer Aided Medical Procedures, March 2008.

[215] T. SIELHORST, M. A. BAUER, O. WENISCH, G. KLINKER, AND N. NAVAB, *Online estimation of the target registration error for n-ocular optical tracking systems*, in Proc. Int'l Conf. Medical Image Computing and Computer Assisted Intervention (MICCAI), 2007. To appear at Int'l Conf. Medical Image Computing and Computer Assisted Intervention (MICCAI).

[216] T. SIELHORST, C. BICHLMEIER, S. M. HEINING, AND N. NAVAB, *Depth perception a major issue in medical ar: Evaluation study by twenty surgeons*, in Proc. Int'l Conf. Medical Image Computing and Computer Assisted Intervention (MICCAI), R. Larsen, M. Nielsen, and J. Sporring, eds., Lecture Notes in Computer Science, 2006.

[217] T. SIELHORST, M. FEUERSTEIN, AND N. NAVAB, *Advanced medical displays: A literature review of augmented reality*, to appear in IEEE/OSA Journal of Display Technology, (2008).

References

[218] T. SIELHORST, M. FEUERSTEIN, J. TRAUB, O. KUTTER, AND N. NAVAB, *Campar: A software framework guaranteeing quality for medical augmented reality*, International Journal of Computer Assisted Radiology and Surgery, 1 (2006), pp. 29–30.

[219] T. SIELHORST, W. SA, A. KHAMENE, F. SAUER, AND N. NAVAB, *Measurement of absolute latency for video see through augmented reality*, in Proc. IEEE and ACM Int'l Symp. on Mixed and Augmented Reality (ISMAR), 2007.

[220] T. SIELHORST, R. STAUDER, M. HORN, T. MUSSACK, A. SCHNEIDER, H. FEUSSNER, AND N. NAVAB, *Simultaneous replay of automatically synchronized videos of surgeries for feedback and visual assessment*, International Journal of Computer Assisted Radiology and Surgery,Supplement 1, 2 (2007), pp. 433–434.

[221] M. SLOMCZYKOWSKI, M. ROBERTO, P. SCHNEEBERGER, C. OZDOBA, AND P. VOCK, *Radiation dose for pedicle screw insertion. Fluoroscopic method versus computer-assisted surgery*, Spine, 24 (1999), pp. 975–983.

[222] E. SPIEGEL, H. T. WYCIS, M. MARKS, AND A. LEE, *Stereotaxic apparatus for operations on the human brain*, Science, 106 (1947), pp. 349–350.

[223] M. W. SPONG, S. HUTCHINSON, AND M. VIDYASAGAR, *Robot Modeling And Control*, John Wiley & Sons, Inc., 2006.

[224] H. STEINHAUS, *Sur la localisation au moyen des rayons x*, Comptes Rendus de L'Academie des Science, 206 (1938), pp. 1473–5.

[225] R. STEINMEIER, R. FAHLBUSCH, O. GANSLANDT, C. NIMSKY, M. BUCHFELDER, M. KAUS, T. HEIGL, G. LENZ, R. KUTH, AND W. HUK, *Intraoperative magnetic resonance imaging with the magnetom open scanner: Concepts, neurosurgical indications, and procedures: A preliminary report*, Neurosurgery Online, 43 (1998), pp. 739–747.

[226] G. D. STETTEN AND V. S. CHIB, *Overlaying ultrasound images on direct vision*, Journal Ultrasound in Medicine, 20 (2001), pp. 235–240.

[227] G. D. STETTEN, A. COIS, W. CHANG, D. SHELTON, R. J. TAMBURO, J. CASTELLUCCI, AND O. VON RAMM, *C-mode real time tomographic reflection for a matrix array ultrasound sonic flashlight*, in Proc. Int'l Conf. Medical Image Computing and Computer Assisted Intervention (MICCAI), R. E. Ellis and T. M. Peters, eds., Lecture Notes in Computer Science, Springer-Verlag, 2003.

[228] J. STIEHL, W. KONERMANN, AND R. HAAKER, eds., *Navigation and Robotics in Total Joint and Spine Surgery*, Springer, 2004.

[229] J. B. STIEHL, W. H. KONERMANN, R. G. HAAKER, AND A. DIGIOIA, eds., *Navigation and MIS in Orthopedic Surgery*, Springer, 2006.

[230] G. STRAUSS, M. FISCHER, J. MEIXENSBERGER, V. FALK, C. TRANTAKIS, D. WINKLER, F. BOOTZ, O. BURGERT, A. DIETZ, AND H. LEMKE, *Bestimmung der effizienz von intraoperativer technologie*, HNO, 54 (2006), pp. 528–535.

[231] M. SYNOWITZ AND J. KIWIT, *Surgeon's radiation exposure during percutaneous vertebroplasty*, J Neurosurg Spine., 4 (2006), pp. 106–109.

[232] R. SZELISKI, *Image alignment and stitching: A tutorial*, tech. report, Microsoft Research, 2006.

[233] J. TALAIRACH AND P. TOURNOUX, *Co-Planar Stereotaxic Atlas of the Human Brain*, Thieme, 1988.

[234] N. THEOCHAROPOULOS, K. PERISINAKIS, J. DAMILAKIS, G. PAPADOKOSTAKIS, A. HADJIPAVLOU, AND N. GOURTSOYIANNIS, *Occupational exposure from common fluoroscopic projections used in orthopaedic surgery*, The Journal of Bone and Joint Surgery (American), 85 (2003), pp. 1698–1703.

[235] J. TRAUB, H. HEIBEL, P. DRESSEL, S. HEINING, R. GRAUMANN, AND N. NAVAB, *A multi-view opto-xray imaging system: Development and first application in trauma surgery*, in Proc. Int'l Conf. Medical Image Computing and Computer Assisted Intervention (MICCAI), 2007.

[236] J. TRAUB, S. KAUR, P. KNESCHAUREK, AND N. NAVAB, *Evaluation of electromagnetic error correction methods*, in Proceedings of BVM 2007, Springer, March 2007.

[237] J. TRAUB, T. SIELHORST, S.-M. HEINING, AND N. NAVAB, *Advanced display and visualization concepts for image guided surgery*, (submitted to) IEEE Journal of Display Technology, (2008).

[238] J. TRAUB, P. STEFAN, S.-M. HEINING, T. SIELHORST, C. RIQUARTS, E. EULER, AND N. NAVAB, *Hybrid navigation interface for orthopedic and trauma surgery*, in Proc. Int'l Conf. Medical Image Computing and Computer Assisted Intervention (MICCAI), R. Larsen, M. Nielsen, and J. Sporring, eds., vol. 4190 of Lecture Notes in Computer Science, Copenhagen, Denmark, Oct. 2006, MICCAI Society, Springer, pp. 373–380.

[239] J. TRAUB, P. STEFAN, S.-M. HEINING, T. SIELHORST, C. RIQUARTS, E. EULER, AND N. NAVAB, *Stereoscopic augmented reality navigation for trauma surgery: cadaver experiment and usability study*, International Journal of Computer Assisted Radiology and Surgery, 1 (2006), pp. 30–31.

[240] J. TRAUB, P. STEFAN, S.-M. HEINING, T. SIELHORST, C. RIQUARTS, E. EULER, AND N. NAVAB, *Towards a hybrid navigation interface: Comparison of a slice based navigation system with in-situ visualization*, in Medical Imaging and Augmented Reality, G.-Z. Yang, T. Jiang, D. Shen, L. Gu, and J. Yang, eds., vol. 4091 of Lecture Notes in Computer Science, Shanghai, China, Aug. 2006, Springer, pp. 179–186.

References

[241] J. TROCCAZ AND P. MERLOZ, *Future Challenges*, vol. Computer and Robotic Assisted Hip and Knee Surgery, Oxford University Press, 2004, ch. 26, pp. 317–326.

[242] R. TSAI, *A versatile camera calibration technique for high accuracy 3d machine vision metrology using off-the-shelf tv cameras and lenses*, IEEE Journal of Robotics and Automation, RA-3 (1987), pp. 323–344.

[243] R. Y. TSAI AND R. K. LENZ, *A new technique for fully autonomous and efficient 3d robotics hand/eye calibration*, IEEE Transactions on Robotics and Automation, 5 (1989), pp. 345–358.

[244] S. UMEYAMA, *Least-squares estimation of transformation parameters between two point patterns*, IEEE Trans. Pattern Anal. Machine Intell., 13 (1991), pp. 376–380.

[245] M. VIERGEVER, ed., *Special Issue on Image Guidance of Therapy*, vol. 17, IEEE Transaction on Medical Imaging, 1998.

[246] S. VOGT, A. KHAMENE, AND F. SAUER, *Reality augmentation for medical procedures: System architecture, single camera marker tracking, and system evaluation*, Int. J. Comput. Vision, 70 (2006), pp. 179–190.

[247] S. VOGT, A. KHAMENE, F. SAUER, AND H. NIEMANN, *Single camera tracking of marker clusters: Multiparameter cluster optimization and experimental verification*, in IEEE and ACM International Symposium on Mixed and Augmented Reality, 2002, pp. 127–136.

[248] F. K. WACKER, S. VOGT, A. KHAMENE, J. A. JESBERGER, S. G. NOUR, D. R. ELGORT, F. SAUER, J. L. DUERK, AND J. S. LEWIN, *An augmented reality system for mr image - guided needle biopsy: Initial results in a swine model*, Radiology, 238 (2006), pp. 497–504.

[249] M. Y. WANG, C. R. MAURER, JR., J. M. FITZPATRICK, AND R. J. MACIUNAS, *An automatic technique for finding and localizing externally attached markers in ct and mr volume images of the head*, IEEE Trans. Biomed. Eng., 43 (1996), pp. 627–637.

[250] C. WARE AND R. BALAKRISHNAN, *Reaching for Objects in VR Displays: Lag and Frame Rate*, ACM Transactions on Computer-Human Interaction, 1 (1994), pp. 331–356.

[251] S. WEBB, ed., *The physics of medical imaging*, Taylor & Francis, 1988.

[252] A. WEIDNER, *Navigation in cervical spine surgery*, in Navigation and Robotics in Total Joint and Spine Surgery, J. B. Stiehl, W. H. Konermann, and R. G. A. Haaker, eds., Springer, 2004, ch. 68, pp. 487–494.

[253] G. WELCH AND E. FOXLIN, *Motion tracking: no silver bullet, but a respectable arsenal*, IEEE Computer Graphics and Applications, 22 (2002), pp. 24–38.

References

[254] T. WENDLER, M. FEUERSTEIN, J. TRAUB, T. LASSER, J. VOGEL, F. DAGHIGHIAN, S. ZIEGLER, AND N. NAVAB, *Real-time fusion of ultrasound and gamma probe for navigated localization of liver metastases*, in Proc. Int'l Conf. Medical Image Computing and Computer Assisted Intervention (MICCAI), N. Ayache, S. Ourselin, and A. Maeder, eds., vol. 4792 of Lecture Notes in Computer Science, Brisbane, Australia, October/November 2007, Springer-Verlag, pp. 252–260.

[255] T. WENDLER, A. HARTL, T. LASSER, J. TRAUB, F. DAGHIGHIAN, S. ZIEGLER, AND N. NAVAB, *Towards intra-operative 3d nuclear imaging: reconstruction of 3d radioactive distributions using tracked gamma probes*, in Proc. Int'l Conf. Medical Image Computing and Computer Assisted Intervention (MICCAI), 2007. To appear at Int'l Conf. Medical Image Computing and Computer Assisted Intervention (MICCAI).

[256] T. WENDLER, J. TRAUB, S. ZIEGLER, AND N. NAVAB, *Navigated three dimensional beta probe for optimal cancer resection*, in Proc. Int'l Conf. Medical Image Computing and Computer Assisted Intervention (MICCAI), R. Larsen, M. Nielsen, and J. Sporring, eds., vol. 4190 of Lecture Notes in Computer Science, Copenhagen, Denmark, Oct. 2006, MICCAI Society, Springer, pp. 561–569.

[257] M. N. WERNICK, *Emission Tomography. The Fundamentals of PET and SPECT*, Academic Press, 2004.

[258] J. B. WEST, J. M. FITZPATRICK, S. A. TOMS, C. R. MAURER, AND R. J. MACIUNAS, *Fiducial point placement and the accuracy of point-based, rigid body registration.*, Neurosurgery, 48 (2001), pp. 810–817.

[259] G. M. WHATLING AND L. D. NOKES, *Literature review of current techniques for the insertion of distal screws into intramedullary locking nails injury*, Injury, 37 (2005), pp. 109–119.

[260] A. WOLBARST, *Physics of radiology*, Medical Physics Publishing, 2nd ed., 2005.

[261] A. WOLBARST AND W. HENDEE, *Evolving and experimental technologies in medical imaging*, Radiology, 238 (2006), pp. 16–39.

[262] Z. YANIV, *Rigid Registration*, Image-Guided Interventions - Technology and Applications, Springer, 2008, ch. 6.

[263] Z. YANIV AND K. CLEARY, *Image-guided procedures: A review*, tech. report, Computer Aided Interventions and Medical Robotics, Imaging Science and Information Systems Center, Department of Radiology, Georgetown University Medical Center, Washington, DC, 20007, USA, April 2006.

[264] Z. YANIV AND L. JOSKOWICZ, *Long bone panoramas from fluoroscopic x-ray images*, IEEE transactions on medical imaging, volume 23; part 1 (2004), pp. 26–35.

References

[265] Z. ZHANG, *Iterative point matching for registration of free-form curves*, Tech. Report 1658, Institut National de Recherche en Informatique et en Automatique (INRIA), 1992.

[266] ——, *A flexible new technique for camera calibration*, IEEE Transactions on Pattern Analysis and Machine Intelligence, 22 (2000), pp. 1330–1334.

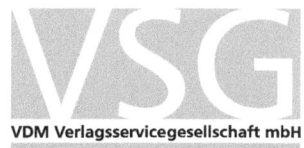

Die VDM Verlagsservicegesellschaft sucht für wissenschaftliche Verlage abgeschlossene und herausragende

Dissertationen, Habilitationen, Diplomarbeiten, Master Theses, Magisterarbeiten usw.

für die kostenlose Publikation als Fachbuch.

Sie verfügen über eine Arbeit, die hohen inhaltlichen und formalen Ansprüchen genügt, und haben Interesse an einer honorarvergüteten Publikation?

Dann senden Sie bitte erste Informationen über sich und Ihre Arbeit per Email an *info@vdm-vsg.de*.

Sie erhalten kurzfristig unser Feedback!

VDM Verlagsservicegesellschaft mbH
Dudweiler Landstr. 99   Telefon +49 681 3720 174
D - 66123 Saarbrücken   Fax   +49 681 3720 1749

www.vdm-vsg.de

Die VDM Verlagsservicegesellschaft mbH vertritt

 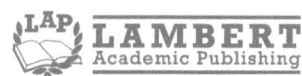 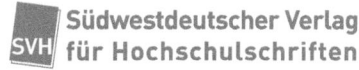

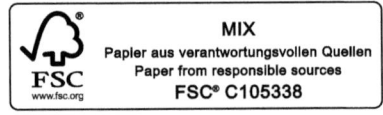

Printed by Books on Demand GmbH, Norderstedt / Germany